"Dr. Carolyn Ross's workbook is a breath of fresh air! Jam-packed with cutting edge information, *The Overcoming Binge Eating and Compulsive Overeating Workbook* helps readers find freedom and health in our weight-obsessed culture. By shedding light on the truth about recovering from binge-eating disorder and compulsive overeating, this book promises to make a real difference in people's lives."

—Jenni Schaefer, author of *Life Without Ed* and *Goodbye Ed, Hello Me*

"Dr. Ross's holistic explanation of binge eating and obesity can change our views of dieting forever. She has lectured to medical and professional audiences about changing our country's dieting mentality. Her wisdom about healing the relationship with food, weight, and body image is presented in a way that finally makes sense. This book can make a difference that can last a lifetime."

—Rebecca Cooper, MA, CCH, CEDS, author of *Diets Don't Work* and founder of Rebecca's House Eating Disorder Treatment Programs

"This is the best practical information I've seen on managing eating disorders. Dr. Carolyn Coker Ross's sound advice can help the many people trapped in destructive relationships to food regain control of their lives and health."

—Andrew Weil, MD, integrative medicine pioneer and author of *Eight Weeks to Optimum Health* and *Healthy Aging*

The Binge Eating & Compulsive Overeating Workbook

An Integrated Approach to Overcoming Disordered Eating

CAROLYN COKER ROSS, MD, MPH

New Harbinger Publications, Inc.

Publisher's Note

This publication is designed to provide accurate and authoritative information in regard to the subject matter covered. It is sold with the understanding that the publisher is not engaged in rendering psychological, financial, legal, or other professional services. If expert assistance or counseling is needed, the services of a competent professional should be sought.

Distributed in Canada by Raincoast Books

Copyright © 2009 by Carolyn Coker Ross, MD, MPH
New Harbinger Publications, Inc.
5674 Shattuck Avenue
Oakland, CA 94609
www.newharbinger.com

Some DBT concepts and exercises in chapter 5 have been adapted for *Skills Training Manual for Treating Borderline Personality Disorder* by Marsha Linehan, © 1993, with permission of the publisher.

Acquired by Melissa Kirk; Cover design by Amy Shoup
Edited by Amy Johnson; Text design by Tracy Marie Carlson

Library of Congress Cataloging-in-Publication Data

Ross, Carolyn Coker.
 The binge eating and compulsive overeating workbook : an integrated approach to overcoming disordered eating / Carolyn Coker Ross.
    p. cm.
 Includes bibliographical references.
 ISBN-13: 978-1-57224-591-4 (pbk. : alk. paper)
 ISBN-10: 1-57224-591-3 (pbk. : alk. paper)
 1. Eating disorders. 2. Eating disorders--Psychological aspects. 3.
 Nutrition. I. Title.
 RC552.E18R67 2009
 616.85'26--dc22

                    2009014667

FSC
Mixed Sources
Product group from well-managed forests and other controlled sources
Cert no. SW-COC-002283
www.fsc.org
© 1996 Forest Stewardship Council

11 10 09

10 9 8 7 6 5 4 3 2 1

First printing

Contents

Introduction 1

Part 1
Healing the Body

CHAPTER 1
What Are Binge Eating and Compulsive Eating? 7

CHAPTER 2
Your Body's Response to Too Much of a Good Thing 11

CHAPTER 3
Understanding Nutrition Basics 19
written with Alicia Trocker, MS, RD

CHAPTER 4
Nourishing Your Body 35
written with Alicia Trocker, MS, RD

PART 2
Healing the Mind

CHAPTER 5

Overview of Traditional Approaches to BED/CO 51

CHAPTER 6

What's Food Got to Do with BED/CO? 65

CHAPTER 7

Mirror, Mirror 79
written with Isabelle Tierney, MA, LMFT, BHSP

CHAPTER 8

Challenging Your Core Beliefs 95

CHAPTER 9

Co-occurring Diagnoses 117
written with Andrew Stropko, Ph.D.

PART 3
Healing the Spirit

CHAPTER 10

Coping with Stress 133

CHAPTER 11

Tools to Manage Stress 145

CHAPTER 12

Nourishing Your Spirit 161

Conclusion: Five Steps to Healing from Eating Disorders 173

Resources 183

References 185

Introduction

Binge eating disorder (BED) and compulsive overeating (CO) are problems that affect millions of people. If you have fought to stop bingeing or overeating, if you have struggled to cope with the emotions that accompany these behaviors, this workbook will help you. You *can* break the vicious cycle of desperation, self-defeating behavior, and negative thinking of BED and CO. This book offers hope and help to all of you who have been frustrated and felt like giving up on yourself because you haven't been able to make your life whole and satisfying on the deepest level possible.

In my thirty years of practice, I have worked with many patients with BED and CO. Indeed, I have worked with women and men just like you—and have been successful in helping many of them change their lives for the better. My training in preventive medicine and public health initially led me to focus on lifestyle behaviors that affect health, such as disordered eating, smoking, and drug and alcohol abuse/dependence. Then, after twenty years of practice, I completed a two-year fellowship in integrative medicine with Dr. Andrew Weil at the University of Arizona. More recently, as the director of an inpatient eating disorder program, I developed a unique integrative medicine approach to treating anorexia, bulimia, binge eating disorder, and compulsive overeating. This integrative approach changed the lives of those I treated. This approach, my training in integrative medicine, and my years of experience are the foundation of this workbook.

The integrative medicine approach I created and share with you in this book combines the best conventional treatments for BED and CO—for example, cognitive therapy, medication, and nutrition—with the use of complementary therapies such as dietary supplements, acupuncture, massage, and others well-supported by research. This approach goes beyond treating symptoms and behaviors to treating underlying root causes. As a result, this book will help you tap into your own body's healing capacity, gain insight into the origin of your disease, and give you the tools and skills you need to transform your life.

This workbook addresses lifestyle elements, nutritional deficits, psychological issues, medical problems, and diagnoses that often accompany BED and CO (such as depression, anxiety, and trauma) using a whole person approach. This will empower you to make the changes I know you want to make—the changes that will help you feel better and be healthier and happier in your life. This book is not about losing weight. Nor is it about looking better in your clothes, although either or both of these may happen. Three decades of working with patients have taught me that happiness and good health are necessary to both feel better and look better. Without the first, the second is impossible.

WHAT THIS BOOK OFFERS YOU

Perhaps you have picked up this book because you're tired of worrying about your appearance or about health issues related to being overweight. You may have fought for some time to stop bingeing or overeating, trying different diets to lose weight, all without long-term success. By now, you've probably had your "fill" of dieting and being told to eat this or not to eat that. You may be concerned about your health or have been told by your physician that your weight is a major health risk. Again, this book is not a diet book. This book will teach you more about the reasons behind your behaviors—and strategies to manage them. This book will help you if:

* You are willing to learn and practice the strategies in this book. Practicing these strategies will enable you to change the behaviors that cause you distress.

* You've decided that you need to change the ways you deal with stress and regulate your emotions, because what you've been doing isn't working.

* You want to dig deeper and find the underlying core beliefs that drive your behaviors.

* You know you want to stop living your life at the mercy of BED and CO.

Whether you are just beginning to think about changing your life or are fully committed to the need to change, this book will provide you with specific skills that, if practiced, can transform your relationships with others and, more importantly, your relationship with your emotions and your body. The exercises and resources in this book will help you focus on the issues that contribute to your BED and CO—and help you begin to make the changes that will put you on the path to full recovery.

HOW THIS BOOK IS DIFFERENT

Conventional medical and psychological approaches to BED and CO focus on managing medical consequences, stopping behaviors, and treating symptoms such as depression or anxiety. Yet despite many medical advances over the past twenty-five years—including numerous new medications for these conditions—very little has changed. Today, many people with BED and CO continue to struggle with yo-yo dieting, poor self-esteem, and serious medical consequences.

This book presents a unique integrative medicine approach to treating BED and CO. *Integrative medicine* is a healing-oriented discipline that takes into account the whole person—body, mind, and spirit—including all aspects of lifestyle. It emphasizes the therapeutic relationship (between you and your treatment team) and makes use of both conventional and alternative therapies. This approach will help you heal on the deepest levels possible.

BOOKMAP: MAPPING THE WORKBOOK

This workbook should be read in the order presented as each section lays the groundwork for the next. Informational sections are intermixed with many self-exploration exercises to help you gain a better understanding of your BED/CO. I suggest you also keep a journal as you proceed through the book.

The arrangement of this workbook reflects the whole person approach I use in working with my patients, with sections on healing the body, mind, and spirit. Part 1 (chapters 1–4) of this workbook focuses on healing the body through lifestyle changes such as nutrition and exercise. Chapter 1 will help you identify whether you have BED or CO; chapter 2 explores the uncertainties inherent in how we measure weight and the medical consequences of BED and CO. Chapters 3 and 4, written with Alicia Trocker, MS, RD, offer basic nutritional information, and help you to evaluate your current diet and assess your individual needs for dietary supplements. Alicia Trocker is an outpatient dietician at UCLA Medical Center, a project coordinator and instructor at UCLA Extension, and a contributing author to the newsletter of UCLA's National Center for Excellence in Women's Health. Alicia lectures at the David Geffen School of Medicine and mentors medical students in developing nonjudgmental nutrition counseling skills.

Part 2 (chapters 5–9) is about healing on the mental or psychological level. Chapter 5 discusses conventional approaches to treating BED and CO, such as cognitive behavioral therapy and medication. Chapters 6 explores what food means to us in a more metaphorical sense, such as "food as love," and how food and mood are connected. In chapter 7, written with Isabelle Tierney, MA, LMFT, BHSP, we focus in depth on the problem of negative body image and how to overcome it. Isabelle Tierney is a licensed marriage and family therapist, a certified Brennan Healing Science therapist, founder of the Body Beloved philosophy—which teaches people to love their bodies from the inside out—and creator and president of The Habit Experts, a company that creates products and services to help people with painful habits. She is also a published writer, workshop leader, and Internet host. Her upcoming book, *The Body Beloved: The Inside-Out Way to Loving Your Body*, serves as the inspiration for this chapter.

In chapter 8, we'll explore the core beliefs that contribute to your eating disorder. Next, in chapter 9, written with Andrew Stropko, Ph.D., we'll discuss mood disorders commonly associated with BED and CO, as well as specific treatments; here you'll learn skills and integrative therapies that can help you interrupt problematic behaviors and change your negative self-talk. Dr. Stropko is the chief psychologist at the prestigious Sierra Tucson, an inpatient hospital located in Tucson, Arizona. A retired lieutenant colonel from the U.S. Army Medical Department, he holds a doctorate from Texas Tech University.

Part 3 (chapters 10–12) focuses on healing the spirit. Chapter 10 explores the impact of stress on disordered eating, while chapter 11 offers tools to better cope with stress so it will no longer control your life. Chapter 12 focuses on ways to nourish your spirit and how to explore your spiritual connectedness. Finally, in the conclusion, I describe five key steps that will empower you to keep moving forward in your recovery from BED/CO.

This workbook is the beginning of your journey to healing. Please use it to its fullest! Make notes, journal, and respond to the exercises. It is my hope that through this process you will find the help you need to become a healthier, happier person.

PART 1

Healing the Body

CHAPTER 1

What Are Binge Eating and Compulsive Eating?

Melinda, a patient, says of her binge eating disorder, "I eat and eat and I know that I should stop, but I can't. I eat so much that I want to throw up, my stomach hurts, and I have to lie down. Sometimes, I feel like if I don't eat everything I can get my hands on, I'll explode." Her words highlight the anguish that many people feel when food controls their lives.

Both binge eating disorder (BED) and compulsive overeating (CO) are conditions in which food is typically used for unhealthy reasons. People with BED or CO tend to feel powerless, and often lose hope that their behavior can change.

WHAT IS BINGE EATING DISORDER?

Binge eating disorder affects between 2 and 5 percent (Spitzer et al. 1993) of adults in the United States (more than four million Americans) and is the most common eating disorder. Up to 25 percent of overweight or obese individuals seeking treatment for obesity have binge eating disorder (Pull 2004). This percentage increases in those who are severely obese. Unlike other eating disorders, binge eating disorder appears to be almost as common in men as it is in women (Grucza, Przybeck, and Cloniger 2007); it affects African Americans as often as Caucasians (Mitchell and Mazzeo 2004).

If you have periods in which you eat large quantities of food in one sitting (the definition of a binge) you may have binge eating disorder. Other symptoms of BED include difficulty in controlling how much you eat and feeling powerless to stop eating, even though you may no longer be hungry or may feel too full. After a binge, you may suffer from emotions of disgust, shame, or embarrassment about your behavior.

For individuals with BED, weight problems are likely to begin earlier than for their peers; often they have a history of obesity, and may have started dieting at a young age (Johnsen et al. 2003). The BED obsession with body shape and size bears a greater similarity to thought patterns of individuals with bulimia nervosa than those of individuals with obesity who don't binge. A hallmark of BED is a history of exposure to negative messages about shape, eating, and weight. While dieting may be associated with BED, in the majority of people, bingeing behavior begins before dieting (Stunkard 2004).

WHAT IS COMPULSIVE OVEREATING?

If you don't fit the criteria for BED, but have struggled with your weight for most of your life, going on and off diets, you may be a compulsive overeater (CO). If so, this book can still help you. The main difference between BED and CO is that people with CO don't experience discrete episodes of binge eating; they tend to eat past the point of fullness, but don't necessarily binge while alone or hide their overeating.

HOW ARE BED AND CO DIFFERENT?

The stories below describe two patients, one with BED, the other with CO:

David, the Compulsive Overeater

David's parents fought constantly when he was growing up. After every fight, David's mother would take him into the kitchen and cook their favorite comfort foods, encouraging David to eat with her. David was overweight as a child, but his mother insisted that he just had "big bones." In college, he played sports and lost weight, but after college the weight came back. David overate when he was happy, sad, or lonely. Although he successfully lost weight on diets, the weight always came back. By the time he was an adult, married with two small children, David's weight was in the obese range and affecting his health. David suffered from depression. He felt he was a failure because he could not control his overeating.

Jennifer, the Binge Eater

Jennifer's mother died when Jennifer was eight. At the time, her father sent her to live with her grandmother, who was very strict and emotionally distant. Here she began to sneak food and binge eat. After gaining weight in middle school, she was put on a strict diet. She was ostracized by the "popular" girls, who often teased her and said mean things about her. At night, Jennifer would sneak downstairs to the kitchen to eat the leftovers. After every episode of bingeing, she felt ashamed and disgusted with herself. In high school, she was diagnosed with depression and put on medication, but couldn't stop bingeing. She felt isolated and alone. She tried to make a fresh start in college, vowing not to binge anymore. But here she felt even more pressure to fit in, and began dieting to lose weight. When she felt fat her whole day was ruined. She knew she should stop but couldn't, often eating to the point of abdominal pain. She felt caught up in a vicious cycle of bingeing and trying not to binge; it was ruining her life.

Both Jennifer and David use food to cope with their emotions; both feel embarrassed and upset with their inability to control their behaviors. Both also often eat when they are not hungry or overeat when they are full. However, Jennifer has specific periods of time when she binges, while David tends to overeat throughout the day. Jennifer's bingeing causes emotional distress and leads to other behaviors to hide it. These behaviors—rooted in the shame, disgust, and guilt she feels about her actions—may create havoc in her life. Of the two, Jennifer is more likely to judge her worth as a person on how she looks or on how she feels about her body than David is.

In comparisons between obese patients who do not have BED and obese patients who do have BED, those with BED tend to have more fluctuation in their weight, experience higher levels of body dissatisfaction (Marcus et al. 1992), and are more likely to have been overweight as a child (Fairburn et al. 1998). Those with BED also have a higher incidence of depression and anxiety (Yanovski 1993). When asked to eat as much as they want in laboratory settings, people with BED will eat significantly more calories than those with CO (Walsh and Boudreau 2003).

Several risk factors for both BED and CO have been identified. These include genetics (which we'll discuss further in chapter 2), low social support, pressure to be thin, emotional eating, depression, low self-esteem (Stice, Presnell, and Spangler 2002), bullying by peers, and some form of maltreatment in childhood (physical or sexual abuse) (Striegel-Moore et al. 2002).

BED currently falls into a diagnostic category called "Eating Disorders Not Otherwise Specified" (EDNOS) in the American Psychiatric Association's *Diagnostic and Statistical Manual* (American Psychiatric Association 2000). EDNOS includes all eating disorders that don't meet criteria for anorexia or bulimia. However, despite sharing many characteristics with other eating disorders, compulsive overeating has thus far not been considered part of the eating disorder spectrum.

WHAT CAUSES BINGE EATING DISORDER AND COMPULSIVE OVEREATING?

There is no known cause for BED or CO. Also unclear is the relationship between dieting and BED, and whether depression causes BED or BED leads to depression. What *is* clear is that skipping meals, eating less than your body needs, and restricting categories of food that are thought to be fattening can lead to overeating or binge eating.

Many people with BED and CO have difficulty expressing their emotions, and may overeat or binge when happy, sad, bored, anxious, or stressed. Those with BED may also abuse alcohol, find it difficult to regulate their emotions (that is, they may feel that their emotions are in charge as opposed to the other way around), or act impulsively. In both BED and CO, social isolation or social withdrawal may occur. Strong genetic links exist for both BED and CO; these disorders may occur in several members of the same family.

Both binge eating disorder and compulsive overeating can serve as ways to cope with emotions, stressful situations, relationship problems, even issues from your childhood. It may be that when you find yourself home alone on a Friday night, food feels like your only reliable friend. Or you may have grown up in a family where dieting and talking about food and weight were part of the daily routine. If you were started on the diet treadmill as a child, you may no longer even know how to get off it. Or perhaps your disordered eating began after a traumatic event, when food soothed a chaos of emotions you didn't know how to handle. No matter what your problems with eating may be, this book will help you develop a healthier relationship with both food and your body.

SUMMARY

Recognizing that you have BED or CO is the first step on your road to recovery. Once you know you have a problem, you've gone a long way toward solving it.

CHAPTER 2

Your Body's Response to Too Much of a Good Thing

If you've struggled with your weight, you may have gotten the message from the health care profession that being overweight causes a laundry list of health problems. It can be frustrating to feel as if you're being told that losing weight is the solution to all your problems—particularly when visiting a medical professional for an issue unrelated to weight. Your medical professional's advice, while technically correct, does not fully address the health consequences of either BED or CO.

In this chapter we will explore how BED, CO, obesity, and behaviors used to control weight—and incidentally to manage emotions—affect your health. But the material in this chapter goes beyond just providing you with simple facts. Instead, it helps you put these facts in perspective. Once in perspective, you will feel less shame and guilt and—most importantly—less self-blame for the situation in which you find yourself.

THE SKINNY ON WEIGHT

First, let's talk about how we measure weight, what these different measurements mean, and how they're used. Once these facts are out of the way, we can focus on how your body works and how to help it work better.

You may be surprised to learn that definitions of obesity and being overweight have varied widely over time. In the past, the Metropolitan Life Insurance Company was the source of standards for weight ranges in the United States and Canada. Currently, body mass index (BMI), waist circumference (WC), and waist-hip ratio (WHR) are the standards used to relate weight to risks for disease and death.

In a moment we will talk a lot about various numbers and what they mean about your individual health risks. However, don't judge yourself as a result of your numbers. This kind of harsh judgment—on scales of any kind—is part of what keeps you trapped in the dieting/bingeing cycle. This self-judgment is something you can change. It's also important to realize that the numbers don't tell the whole story. In fact, many of the cut-offs that physicians use are arbitrary and are only meant to serve as guidelines for understanding how weight affects health risk. What the numbers don't tell you is that even the most rigorous studies haven't looked at the possibility that you can improve your health no matter what size you are.

Body Mass Index

One of the most commonly used measures of overweight is the *body mass index* (BMI). BMI is considered a good measure of body fat, which is used to determine health risk. Here is how to calculate your body mass index:

$$BMI = [\text{your weight in pounds} \div (\text{your height in inches})^2] \times 703$$

The 703 in the formula is used to convert from pounds/inches^2 to kilograms/meters^2.

Next, let's follow a fictional woman and man through the various measurements of weight and see how they fare.

SALLY AND NOAH AND THEIR BMIs

Sally is a thirty-five-year-old Caucasian women who is 5'4" tall. She exercises regularly and describes herself as chunky. Her weight is currently 169 pounds. Noah is a twenty-nine-year-old African American who says that he has been overweight since childhood. He is 6'2" and presently weighs 190 pounds.

Sally's BMI would thus be:

$$BMI = [169 \div (64)^2] \times 703 = 29.0 \text{ kg/m}^2$$

Similarly, Noah's BMI would be:

$$BMI = [190 \div (74)^2] \times 703 = 24.4 \text{ kg/m}^2$$

(We'll return to Sally and Noah in a moment.)

Interpretation of BMI

BMI is influenced by both age and race. At the same BMI, an older person will have more body fat and less muscle than someone who is younger. In addition, the optimal BMI for adults varies by race: for example, it's 23 to 25 for Caucasians and 23 to 30 for African Americans (Fontaine et al. 2003). In

Mexicans surveyed in the Mexican National Survey (Sanchez-Castillo et al. 2003), the risk for diabetes and high blood pressure increased at BMI levels of approximately 26.3 to 27.4 kg/m^2 in men and 27.7 to 28.9 kg/m^2 in women. For Chinese, the risks for high blood pressure and heart disease factors like high cholesterol and diabetes increase at a BMI of 23.8 kg/m^2; and for Japanese, a BMI of greater than or equal to 25 kg/m^2 is associated with twice the risk of high blood pressure than a BMI of 22 kg/m^2 (Bell, Adair, and Popkin 2003). These differences stem primarily from variance in body shape. For example, Asians who become overweight tend to carry their weight in the abdomen, leading to the body shape most associated with heart disease, diabetes, and high blood pressure risk. (We'll discuss this in more detail when we talk about waist circumference.)

Obesity as a young adult has a much greater impact on your health risks than obesity later in life. For example, research suggests that for African Americans older than sixty, being overweight or moderately obese does not affect overall longevity. However, severe obesity at any age is associated with a shortened lifespan in all ethnicities. Because there is currently a paucity of research that conclusively correlates BMI and health risks in different ethnic groups (Fontaine et al. 2003), the medical community in the United States commonly uses the BMI ranges listed in the following table.

BMI Ranges

BMI	Weight Status
Below 18.5	Underweight
18.5–24.9	Normal
25.0–29.9	Overweight
30.0 and above	Obese

Based on these ranges, Sally's BMI of 29.0 would be considered within optimal range if she is African American but not if she's Caucasian. If she's Caucasian she would be considered overweight. As either a Caucasian or an African American, Noah's BMI of 24.4 would be considered normal, but not if he were Chinese.

BMI is a good approximation of body fat but it has some limitations:

* At the same BMI, women have more body fat than men

* At the same BMI, older people on average tend to have more body fat than younger people, so their BMI may not accurately reflect their level of body fat

* Athletes have a high BMI because they are more muscular, not because they have more body fat

Because the relationship between level of body fat and health risk is continuous, the BMI cutoffs for being overweight or obese are somewhat arbitrary. In other words, it's not as if there's a sharp jump in health risk when you cross the line from one category to the next. If you have a BMI of 29, your health risks do not automatically increase if your BMI increases to 30.

Your BMI is not the sole criterion for assessing your personal risk for heart disease or stroke or other health risks. It should only be considered in conjunction with an assessment of other risk factors, including family history and lifestyle factors such as level of activity, diet, and whether or not you smoke. Indeed, researchers are finding that overweight and obese individuals—people with high BMIs—who engage in regular physical activity have reduced health risks when compared to normal weight persons who do not exercise regularly (Blair and Brodney 1999; Bacon et al. 2002). Unfortunately, the medical profession's current focus on the "war on obesity," has led many health care providers—as well as health insurance companies—to use BMI without referencing it to other risk factors.

Calculate Your Body Mass Index

$$BMI = [\text{your weight in pounds} \div (\text{your height in inches})^2] \times 703$$

1. Start with your weight in pounds: _____ .

2. What is your height in inches? (For example, if you're 5'7", that's (5 X 12) + 7 = 67 inches.): _____ .

3. Next, multiply your height in inches by itself (for example if your height is 67 inches multiply 67 X 67): _____ .

4. Divide your weight in pounds by the number you found in step 3 (for example, if your weight is 200 lbs and you're 5'7", that would be 200 ÷ 4,489, or .0446): _____ .

5. Finally, multiply this number by 703 to convert from pounds/inches^2 to kilograms/meters^2: _____ . This is your BMI. (In our example, this would be .0446 X 703, producing a BMI of 31.4)

Your BMI = _____

Your BMI puts you in this category (circle one):

Underweight   Normal   Overweight   Obese

Waist Circumference

Waist circumference (WC) is very helpful as an *independent* (alone or by itself) predictor of risk for certain medical conditions (Lemieux et al. 1996). In particular, it is very useful for predicting abdominal fat—the type of body fat that causes insulin resistance and has an even stronger correlation with health risks than BMI. WC has been found to be a better predictor of health risk than waist-hip ratio (Albu et al. 1997).

Health risks increase for women with a WC greater than 35 inches and for men with a WC greater than 40 inches. (A word of caution: waist circumference may not accurately predict health risks in older people as height loss may increase WC measurements even though body fat has remained the same (Visscher et al. 2001). WC may also underestimate health risks in Asians, who tend to have more body fat at lower levels of both WC and BMI (Wildman et al. 2004). Although WC is an important independent predictor, both WC and BMI predict health risks better when used together than alone.

Waist Circumference

Waist Circumference	MEN	WOMEN
Optimal	35 inches	32.5 inches
Increased health risks	40 inches	35 inches

Individuals with a larger waist circumference tend to have an apple body type—that is, they carry most of their fat deposits in their waist area. Those with a pear body type, on the other hand, carry most of their fat deposits in their hips. Apple body types tend to be at higher risk for heart disease and diabetes. As a result, it is important to place less emphasis on your weight and more emphasis on where you carry your weight.

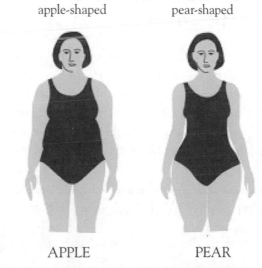

apple-shaped   pear-shaped

APPLE   PEAR

(Photo courtesy of www.womenshealth.gov/faq/weightloss.htm)

Thus, if you are overweight and/or obese but carry your weight in your hips, your health risks will—up to a point—be lower than someone who has the same BMI but who carries weight in the abdomen.

Determine Your Waist Circumference

Wrap a tape measure around your waist at the level of your belly button. Keeping the tape measure parallel to the floor, read the result. This number is your waist circumference (WC): _____ .

Currently, your waist circumference falls into the following category (circle one):

OPTIMAL   INCREASED HEALTH RISKS

SALLY AND NOAH AND WAIST CIRCUMFERENCE

Sally's WC is 34, slightly larger than optimal but less than the 35 inches that marks an increase in health risks. Noah's WC, on the other hand, is 41, falling into the category of increased health risk. Let's summarize our findings for Sally and Noah:

Sally: BMI in the overweight range

WC greater than 32.5 (optimal) but less than 35 (increased health risks)

Noah: BMI in the normal range

WC high, indicating increased health risks

WHAT DOES ALL THIS MEAN?

Although her WC doesn't indicate any problems, according to her BMI measurement, Sally's health risks are increased. With Noah it is the reverse: his BMI falls in the normal range, but his WC—the more important factor in terms of predicting potential for health risks—is high, indicating increased health risks. As a result, it's important that Noah look for ways to reduce his risks, for example, through diet and exercise. For Sally, with a slightly larger than optimal waist circumference, if she has risk factors for heart disease and diabetes other than her weight, she should focus on ways to reduce risks.

Your Summary of Weight and Waist Measures

What about you? Summarize your weight measures below. You can use this information to track your progress over time.

1. Your BMI measurement shows that you are (circle one):

*   Underweight

*   Average

*   Overweight

*   Obese

2. Your waist circumference category is:

*   Optimal

*   Increased health risks

Regardless of your BMI and waist circumference measurement, not all of your risk factors are under your control—as you'll see in the next section.

GENETICS AND BED/CO

Binge eating disorder runs in families; it is estimated that 57 percent of the risk for BED is inherited or genetic (Javaras et al. 2008). Genetics also accounts for 40 to 70 percent of an individual's risk of developing obesity (Stunkard, Harris et al. 1990).

Even though genetics may increase your risk of developing BED or CO, it does not explain certain factors. Why has obesity increased in the U.S. over the last fifty years when the population's genes have not substantially changed? This is in large part because a genetic vulnerability to obesity has collided with increasing access to food as well as greater consumption of foods that are less than healthy.

Many individuals who suffer from BED and CO have been made to feel as if it is their fault they have difficulty losing weight or changing their behaviors. This, as you probably know all too well, isn't helpful. More important is to commit to good health and do whatever you realistically can—in partnership with your health care provider—to become the healthiest that you can, given your genetic makeup.

THE FACTS ABOUT YOUR HEALTH RISKS

It won't be news to you that if you suffer from BED or CO, your risk for certain diseases may be increased. Most of these risks are thought to be related to weight, but may instead be related to overall level of fitness, as little of the research in this area has included individuals who are both overweight and physically fit. These risks include higher probabilities for heart disease, diabetes, high blood pressure, gallstones, and osteoarthritis.

Interestingly, individuals who engage in yo-yo dieting or weight cycling are more likely to suffer from high blood pressure (Brownell and Rodin 1994) and may have reduced immunity (Shade et al. 2004) than obese persons who don't diet at all. Another significant risk for those with BED/CO who are also obese is metabolic syndrome, a constellation of symptoms including high blood pressure, high blood sugar, elevated cholesterol (with low levels of HDL or good cholesterol and high levels of LDL or bad cholesterol), high triglycerides (another fat in our blood), and an increased waist circumference. Individuals with BED/CO who are obese may also suffer from sleep apnea, a condition in which breathing stops during sleep—sometimes for minutes at a time—due to a narrowing of the airway. Sleep apnea may cause heart disease, headaches, weight gain, and memory problems, and is considered a risk factor for diabetes and metabolic syndrome (WebMD 2008).

SUMMARY

Making a commitment to your health is an important beginning step. If you let it, it can motivate you to seek and maintain a strong recovery program.

CHAPTER 3

Understanding Nutrition Basics

written with Alicia Trocker, MS, RD

Let's turn now to nutrition. Understanding the basics of good nutrition can seem difficult given the many different diet recommendations out there. But good nutrition doesn't have to be hard. This chapter will challenge your misconceptions, help you restore your relationship with food, and empower you to follow your own body's guidance to help you choose foods that are nourishing.

The past several decades have seen many changes in nutrition recommendations. These changes have been confusing, often conflicting with each other. This is in part because over the past fifty years we have relied more on results of nutritional research to tell us how to eat—in order to avoid cancer, heart disease, and other chronic diseases—than at any other time in our history. Unfortunately, these scientific recommendations seem to change every few years as new studies point to different nutrients as the cause of diseases. This has led us to shift our understanding of food as nourishing, appetizing, and part of the social fabric of our lives to food as a collection of specific components. For example, at different times fat has been regarded as the cause of all ills, leading to the advent of low-fat diets and food products. Next, carbohydrates were in the national spotlight, first as the most beneficial of foods and then increasingly as the cause of obesity and other medical problems. However, neither the focus on fats nor the focus on carbohydrates has decreased the level of obesity in the United States and other western countries. How can the United States, a nation that is so diet conscious, also be so overweight?

Two factors contribute to our culture's increase in food issues: first, confusion as to what is actually nutritious as a result of these changing and often conflicting scientific recommendations; and second, disturbing trends in modern eating habits.

NUTRITION CONFUSION

A good example of how nutrition recommendations focused on specific components of food may change dramatically is the case of cooking oils. Not very long ago, corn oil was considered the preferred cooking oil. Now, however, we know that polyunsaturated fats such as corn oil oxidize more easily when heated and can be toxic to our bodies. These oxidized fats can then cause free radical damage to our cells, contributing to the development of chronic illnesses such as cancer and heart disease. Nutrition scientists now recommend the use of olive oil for light sautéing and canola oil for frying, because these oils contain primarily monounsaturated fats and are more stable when heated.

Because food science is constantly changing, to develop healthy eating habits you will have to look to a higher source than science—your own body's wisdom and intuition.

DISTURBING TRENDS IN THE MODERN DIET

Two disturbing trends in the modern diet are also contributing to our culture's food issues: our reliance on packaged prepared foods high in partially hydrogenated fats and the extensive use of high fructose corn syrup. These trends, along with a lack of physical exercise, have resulted in the current obesity epidemic in our country.

Processed/Convenience Food

Convenience food—packaged food, fast food, or restaurant food—is a mainstay of the U.S. diet. However, convenience foods are problematic as they make it harder for us to control what is in the food we eat and how much of it we consume. Over time, this has alienated us from our intuitive understanding of how much food we need and whether food is nourishing us or not. This often translates into larger portions to give patrons "extra" value. A patient once asked Alicia, "Why *wouldn't* you super-size a meal, if it's only fifty cents extra?" She replied, "How much more are you spending on larger clothes and doctor bills?" There is a cost beyond that fifty cents; you just don't see it at the time.

With an increased availability of processed foods came the use of partially hydrogenated fats—also known as *trans fats*—which have recently been identified as contributing to increased risk for many chronic diseases. Originally used to extend the shelf life of processed foods, partially hydrogenating a fat involves whipping a liquid fat and adding hydrogen to it until it becomes a solid. In the process, healthy fatty acids are removed. What is left is a product that, when ingested, is likely to raise harmful cholesterol (LDL) and lower protective cholesterol (HDL). Now, most food manufacturers are eliminating trans fats. However, just because a product's label says it contains no trans fats does not guarantee that healthy fats have been used instead.

High Fructose Corn Syrup

The second disturbing trend in our modern diet is our reliance on high fructose corn syrup (HFCS), a cheaper and sweeter alternative to sugar. HFCS is found in non-diet soft drinks and numerous processed foods, including cookies, cake, and candy. Because it is ubiquitous, it is very hard to avoid. Between 1970 and 1990, U.S. consumption of HFCS increased over 1000 percent; currently 40 percent of the sweeteners added to our foods and beverages come from HFCS (Bray, Nielsen, and Popkin 2004). This increase parallels our country's increase in obesity.

When we eat processed sugars rather than natural sugars—such as those in fruit and vegetables—we lose the nutritional value and fiber that would normally both cue our bodies that we are full and can stop eating, and prevent a rapid spike in blood sugar.

There are two important types of sugar: fructose and glucose. *Fructose* is very sweet and found in fruits. In its natural fruit form, fructose is much less concentrated than the HFCS currently added to so many of our foods. (Despite some manufacturers' claims, HFCS is not "natural"—it is corn gone bad. Consumption of it should be avoided or markedly reduced whenever possible.) *Glucose* is what our food is broken down into and is the energy that powers our cells; glucose is what diabetics measure when they test their blood sugar. Our bodies' response to fructose is very different from its response to glucose; when fructose is metabolized in the liver, it tends to go directly to making and storing fat (Bray, Nielsen, and Popkin 2004). All of these elements contribute to overeating and bingeing if you have BED/CO.

HEALTHY EATING

In a moment we'll discuss five very straightforward principles for healthy eating. These five principles will help you slowly and gradually make any necessary changes to your eating habits without the physical trauma of quickly gaining or losing weight and without the emotional trauma of failing at yet another fad diet. First, however, use the following exercise to evaluate your current eating habits.

Your Current Eating Habits

Use the following statements to assess your current eating habits:

1. I eat three meals on most days.   Yes   No

2. I only eat when I am hungry.   Yes   No

3. I rarely skip meals.   Yes   No

4. I eat vegetables two to three times a day.   Yes   No

5. I frequently feel bloated.   Yes   No

6. I eat convenience food three or more times a week.   Yes   No

7. I eat fried food more than once a week.   Yes   No

8. I feel "foggy" and have trouble thinking, especially in the afternoons.   Yes   No

9. I often have headaches.   Yes   No

10. I am often constipated, gassy, or have diarrhea.   Yes   No

11. My weight is stable and does not change by more than a few pounds.   Yes   No

12. I frequently crave certain foods.   Yes   No

If you agreed with statements 1–4 and disagreed with statements 5–12, your eating habits are ideal. If not, please read on.

Principle One: No Food Is Bad Food

Our relationship with food is very complex. Very early in childhood we learn what we like and don't like. Much of this has to do with what our family exposes us to. If you grew up eating a lot of meat and potatoes, you may be upholding the family tradition. The culture in which you were raised also influences food choices. For example, in some parts of the United States, many foods are fried and huge portion sizes are common.

If you've struggled with BED and CO, you may have some skewed beliefs about foods you should and shouldn't eat. Many if not most of these beliefs are probably false. Use the following exercise to challenge these beliefs.

Good vs. Bad Food

Rate the foods below as good or bad, depending on whether you think each food is healthy for you:

Shrimp   Good   Bad

Fried chicken   Good   Bad

Butter   Good   Bad

Potatoes   Good   Bad

Peanut butter   Good   Bad

Beans   Good   Bad

Chocolate   Good   Bad

Ice cream   Good   Bad

Avocados   Good   Bad

List three reasons why you consider bad foods "bad:"

1. _____

2. _____

3. _____

List three reasons why you consider good foods "good:"

1. _____

2. _____

3. _____

Review what's really good and bad about these foods with the following table:

Good vs. Bad Food

Food	What's Good About It	What's Bad About It
Shrimp	Shrimp contains selenium, zinc, B vitamins, iron, and omega-3 fatty acids. Shrimp also helps reduce fatigue and improves conversion of food to energy.	Although high in cholesterol, shrimp is low in saturated fat and total fat content, and therefore doesn't raise blood cholesterol. However, frying or sautéing shrimp in butter will increase both fat and cholesterol content.
Fried chicken	Chicken (fried or otherwise prepared) contains protein, B vitamins, and iron. In addition, chicken broth has been found helpful in treating colds.	Fried chicken has 2–3 times the saturated fat of chicken that has been baked or broiled.
Butter	Butter contains vitamins A and E, calcium, and selenium. Butter helps foster the growth of good bacteria in the gut and may protect against cancer (Aro et al. 2000). Butter also contributes to the production of sex hormones (estrogen, testosterone, progesterone).	Butter is high in saturated fat and cholesterol. Also, when not organic, butter may contain pesticides, growth hormones, and antibiotics.

Potatoes	Potatoes contain potassium, magnesium, zinc, B vitamins, and vitamin C. Moreover, potatoes help reduce high blood pressure, and have virus-fighting and anticancer benefits.	When fried, potatoes can be high in saturated fat. Thus, the recommended serving size of french fries is ten fries. Also, if you have diabetes, you may need to limit your intake of potatoes in order to keep your blood sugar stable.
Peanut butter	Peanut butter is rich in almost all minerals; it contains protein, copper, magnesium, iron, potassium, and B vitamins.	Many popular brands of peanut butter also include hydrogenated oils, salt, and sugar. Peanuts not purchased from a reputable source may be tainted with a carcinogenic mold. Finally, peanuts are a common allergen.
Beans	Beans are an excellent, low-fat source of protein. They contain calcium, magnesium, iron, and potassium, and promote heart health, strong bones, and weight loss.	Although beans are carbohydrates as well as proteins, they are complex carbs, and so do not cause the high spikes in blood sugar and insulin that simple carbs do. However, beans can cause flatulence (gas) in people not accustomed to eating them regularly; over time, this will disappear.
Chocolate	Chocolate with cocoa solids of 60 percent or greater is high in mood enhancers; in addition, chocolate can trigger the release of endorphins. Dark chocolate in particular is also high in antioxidants.	Chocolate treats are typically high in sugar (which can cause spikes in blood sugar) and saturated fat. White chocolate isn't actually chocolate, and so contains no beneficial cocoa solids.
Ice cream	Ice cream contains calcium, vitamin D, and conjugated linoleic acid (an essential fatty acid with cancer-fighting benefits).	Ice cream is high in saturated fat, with some premium brands containing almost twice the amount of saturated fat as others. Thus, the recommended serving size for ice cream is ½ cup. And although ice cream is a source of calcium, it also contains 1½ to 2 times the amount of carbohydrates (sugar) as whole milk, which can cause spikes in blood sugar.

Avocadoes	Avocadoes are rich in heart-healthy monounsaturated fats, potassium, magnesium, calcium, and folic acid as well as vitamins A, D, and E. Eating avocadoes may reduce the risk of heart disease, cancer, and osteoporosis, and lower blood pressure.	Although avocadoes are mostly fat—and as such shouldn't be considered a vegetable in your meal plan—the fat they contain is a healthy fat.

Although some have more nutritional value than others, every one of the foods listed above contributes something different to your overall health and well-being. Of course, eating anything—even something healthy—in excessive quantities or to the exclusion of all else is unhealthy. The purpose of the exercise is for you to identify the judgments you've come to make about food so you can begin to shift your relationship with it. One of the most important choices you can make for good health is to eat a variety of foods.

As someone with BED or CO, you may have developed a very shortsighted view of food that centers on whether it is fattening or high in calories. It can be very liberating to eliminate labels and judgments and just see what your body really wants and needs to feel good.

Principle Two: Eat Fresh and Naked

Fresh food is typically lower in saturated fats, sodium, and sugar than convenience food, and contains greater nutritional value. Nutrients in fresh fruits and vegetables can help lower your risk of heart disease. These nutrients include antioxidant vitamins, potassium (in bananas, oranges, tomatoes), dietary fiber, folate (in dark-green leafy vegetables and beans), and flavonoids (in apples, berries, and onions) (Hu and Cho 2003). In very large studies, people who ate more fruits and vegetables were less likely to have strokes (Gillman et al. 1995), especially if they consumed more cruciferous vegetables (broccoli, cabbage, brussels sprouts), citrus fruit and juices, and vitamin C–rich fruits and vegetables (Kushi, Lenart, and Willett 1995). Vegetables that are rich in carotenoids (vitamin A), such as carrots, broccoli, spinach, yellow squash, tomatoes, and lettuce, may also decrease the risk of coronary artery disease, a narrowing of the blood vessels that supply blood and oxygen to the heart due to cholesterol deposits (Liu et al. 2000).

Another reason to eat fresh food rather than convenience food is that processing can substantially reduce a food's nutrients. For example, during the canning process food loses one-third of many of its vitamins, including A, C, riboflavin, and thiamin. If you can't eat fresh foods, your next best option is frozen vegetables and fruits. Short of that, canned vegetables are better than no vegetables.

Naked foods are those that are in their natural state, without sauces, preservatives, or other additives. Naked foods give you the full, unadulterated benefit of the food. An example of naked foods is nuts; these are best eaten raw and unsalted. Research has found that individuals who eat nuts five or more times a week have lower risks for coronary artery disease than those who rarely eat nuts (Hu and Stampfer 1999) and a lower risk for heart attacks. Further, women who eat nuts and peanut butter are less likely to have type 2 diabetes (Jiang et al. 2002). Although nuts are considered fats, the fat they contain is a healthy one: researchers have found that a diet high in peanuts, walnuts, or almonds lowers LDL (bad) cholesterol (Kris-Etherton et al. 2001). Eating a small handful of nuts a day is a healthy choice.

The more nutrients you obtain from high quality foods, the lower quantities of food you will need to eat to supply your body's nutritional needs.

Principle Three: Your Gut Is Your Ally—Repopulate It

The gastrointestinal tract digests food, absorbing nutrients through the action of billions of bacteria and other microorganisms. *Probiotics* are foods or dietary supplements that contain "good" bacteria or microorganisms similar to those naturally present in the intestinal tract. These microorganisms have anti-inflammatory properties, help maintain our immunity, and may help reduce risks for cancer (Sanders 2000). Probiotics may reduce the severity of chronic constipation (Koebnick et al. 2003) and can reduce gas, bloating, abdominal pain, and cramping in those with irritable bowel syndrome (Kajander, Hatakka, and Poussa 2005). Probiotics may also play a role in preventing colon cancer (Wollowski, Rechkemmer, and Pool-Zobel 2001). Consumption of foods containing these good bacteria may reduce inflammation, thereby reducing the risk of diseases associated with the inflammatory response, such as atherosclerosis, rheumatoid arthritis, and inflammatory bowel diseases (ulcerative colitis, Crohn's disease). Probiotics may also improve the absorption of important minerals.

Recently, researchers have found a relationship between certain gut bacteria and obesity. Two types of gut bacteria were found to be low in obese individuals, increasing with weight loss. These bacteria are thought to affect the body's ability to extract energy from food. Not being able to get enough nutrition/ energy out of your food because your digestive system is not functioning well may contribute to obesity (Turnbaugh et al. 2006).

Two of the most common gut bacteria are *Bifidobacterium* and *Lactobacillus*. Food sources of probiotics include kefir, yogurt, sauerkraut, and kimchi (a pickled or fermented cabbage dish common in Korean meals). A note of caution: high consumption of kimchi has been linked to an increased risk for stomach cancer, so it should not be eaten in excess (Lee et al. 1995). Individuals with BED/CO should include probiotics from food or as a supplement to improve digestive function and the absorption of important nutrients from the diet.

Principle Four: Maximize Your Nutrition with Supplements

The following discussion focuses on basic nutritional supplements you should consider taking. In later chapters we'll discuss supplements used to treat depression and anxiety as well as supplements for managing stress. (The general information in the following sections has been adapted from fact sheets from the Office of Dietary Supplements, part of the National Institutes of Health.)

MULTIVITAMINS

Approximately 64 percent of men and 53 percent of women take multivitamins. However, women who are obese are much less likely to consider taking a multivitamin important for their health (Kimmons 2006). Although multivitamins should not be used in place of food, multivitamins can alleviate a variety of vitamin deficiency and absorption problems. This is particularly important for a number of reasons: 1) recent research has shown more vitamin deficiencies than expected, especially for vitamin D; 2) our food supply is inconsistent in vitamin content due to farming practices that cause soil nutrient depletion; 3) our ability to absorb vitamins decreases with age; and 4) many medications affect the absorption of vitamins (for example, medications used to treat ulcers, acid reflux/GERD, diabetes, high blood pressure, and inflammation). Yet another good reason to take a multivitamin is that multivitamins may also help reduce the incidence of infection (Barringer et al. 2003).

When you purchase a multivitamin look for vitamin A in the form of beta-carotene or mixed carotenoids. Also, unless you are a menstruating woman or your doctor recommends iron, choose a multivitamin without iron.

ESSENTIAL FATTY ACIDS

Essential fatty acids (EFAs) cannot be synthesized by the body and must be obtained through diet or supplementation. There are two types of essential fatty acids: omega-3 and omega-6. The diet of early humans is thought to have included equal amounts of omega-3 fatty acids and omega-6 fatty acids. Now, however, in the West we typically consume ten times more omega-6 fatty acids than omega-3 fatty acids. Linoleic and arachidonic acids, the omega-6 fatty acids most prevalent in the Western diet, promote inflammation, which is thought to be the basis for many chronic diseases such as heart disease, cancer, asthma, arthritis, and depression. (Linoleic acid can also be beneficial; it can be converted in the body to gamma-linoleic acid, which is a healthy omega-6 fatty acid beneficial for skin and hair health.)

Omega-3 fatty acids. The important components of omega-3 fatty acids include eicosapentaenoic acid (EPA) and docosahexaenoic acid (DHA) found in fish (salmon, tuna, halibut) and fish oils, and alpha-linoleic acid (ALA) which is found in seeds and seed oils (flaxseed), walnuts and walnut oil, soybeans, and marine life such as algae and krill.

Omega-3 fatty acids help raise beneficial HDL cholesterol levels, lower blood pressure in persons with high blood pressure (Breslow 2006), and prevent heart disease (Hu and Cho 2003) and stroke (He , Rimm, and Merchant 2002). They may also reduce some of the causes of metabolic syndrome (Ebbesson et al. 2005) and assist overweight individuals in losing weight. Omega-3 fatty acids are used to treat osteoarthritis and inflammatory conditions such as rheumatoid arthritis (Cleland et al. 2006), and can help improve bone density and prevent bone loss, thereby reducing the risk for osteoporosis. Dieting, however, can lead to low levels of essential fatty acids (Bruinsma and Taren 2000).

Omega-3 fatty acids are also lower in individuals with depression (Colin, Reggers, and Castronovo 2003); as a result, omega-3 supplementation may reduce symptoms of depression (Logan 2004). Other conditions that may be helped by omega-3 fatty acids include inflammatory bowel disease (Dichi et al. 2000), asthma, anorexia nervosa (Holman, Adams, and Nelson 1995), and menstrual pain (Deutch 1995). Finally, omega-3 fatty acids may also reduce the risk of developing cancers of the breast, colon, and prostate (Aronson et al. 2001; de Deckere 1999; Lockwood et al. 1994).

MAGNESIUM

Magnesium is important for muscle function, immune system support, nerve function, and maintaining a regular heart rhythm. It is also important for keeping blood pressure normal. Higher blood levels of magnesium may reduce your risk of heart disease. Magnesium may also influence the release of insulin, which controls blood sugar; diabetics often have low blood levels of magnesium. Low levels of magnesium can affect the amount of calcium in bones; however, consumption of magnesium strengthens bones.

Magnesium deficiency can be caused by taking diuretics (water pills), certain antibiotics (Amphotericin and Gentamicin), and certain cancer medications (Cisplatin). Individuals at risk for magnesium deficiency include alcoholics, people with inadequately controlled diabetes, older adults, and those with chronic malabsorption problems (for example, as a result of Crohn's disease, intestinal surgery, or gluten sensitivity).

Magnesium is found in fish, nuts, beans, green leafy vegetables, peanut butter, yogurt, oatmeal, cereal, avocados, bananas, and milk.

VITAMIN D AND CALCIUM

Vitamin D and calcium support bone health; supplementation may reduce the risk of developing osteoporosis (Tang et al. 2007) or osteopenia (low bone density, the precursor to osteoporosis), which affect millions of Americans. Osteoporosis is a major cause of disability from fractures and chronic pain, and can lead to death. Inadequate calcium and vitamin D levels may also increase risks for type 1 and 2 diabetes (Pittas 2007), and may be associated with increased risks for cancer (Lappe et al. 2007; Garland, Garland, and Gorham 2006; Kampman et al. 2000; Chan et al. 2001). On the other hand, higher levels of vitamin D are associated with reduced risk of death from any cause (Autier and Gandini 2007). Obese individuals typically have levels of vitamin D more than 50 percent lower than those of non-obese individuals, because fatty tissue stores vitamin D, making it less available to other body cells (Wortsman et al. 2000). Low levels of calcium and vitamin D are associated with high blood pressure (Scragg, Sowers, and Bell 2007; Allender et al. 1996) and multiple sclerosis (Kampman, Wilsgaard, and Mellgren 2007).

Few foods naturally contain vitamin D. However, many foods are fortified with vitamin D including milk, margarine, and some ready-to-eat cereals, fruit juices, and yogurt. Vitamin D is also produced by the effect of ultraviolet sunshine on the skin.

Dietary sources of calcium include milk, yogurt, cheese, tofu, tuna, salmon, calcium-fortified juices and soy milk, egg yolks, dark-green leafy vegetables, ricotta cheese, and, to a lesser degree, broccoli and whole grain bread.

B VITAMINS

The B vitamins are important in nerve cell health, prevention of birth defects, and immune system support. They are also important to the production of neurotransmitters such as serotonin and dopamine, which affect mood and mental functioning. Researchers have recently found that vitamin B_{12} deficiencies are much more prevalent than expected in individuals over the age of twenty-six (Tucker et al. 2000). Deficiency may result from poor absorption of B vitamins from foods. Certain prescription medications may decrease B-vitamin absorption, including birth control pills, the diabetic drug Metformin, and medications used to treat ulcers or acid reflux. Strict vegetarians who do not eat any animal products may be B-vitamin deficient, as may individuals who have undergone a partial removal of their stomach, and those with celiac disease or Crohn's disease.

Researchers have found that B vitamins may reduce the risk of dementia (Hutto 1997); cancer, including breast and cervical cancer, (Jennings 1995; Choi 1999; Webster 1998); and cataracts (Cumming,

Mitchell, and Smith 2000). B-vitamin supplementation may reduce symptoms of osteoarthritis (Jonas, Rapoza, and Blair 1996) and may improve response to antidepressant medications (Coppen and Bailey 2000). (We'll discuss the use of B vitamins in treating depression in greater detail in chapter 9.)

B vitamins are found in a wide array of foods, including fortified breakfast cereals, fish, pork, chicken, bananas, beans, peanut butter, dark-green leafy vegetables, and many other vegetables.

Supplement Dosages and Cautions

Supplement	Additional Details	Dose	Cautions
Omega-3 Fatty Acids	Look for an omega-3 fatty acid preparation that contains approximately equal amounts of DHA and EPA.	A good starting dose for health maintenance is one gram of combined DHA/EPA daily. For depression, doses can range from 1–3 grams. Higher doses are used in bipolar disorder, but this should be done only under the supervision of your physician.	Omega-3 fatty acids theoretically increase the effects of blood-thinners such as coumadin, aspirin, and Plavix. Taking more than 3 grams per day may deplete vitamin E, so look for an omega-3 product that contains vitamin E, or take vitamin E in a multivitamin.
Magnesium	(None.)	350 milligrams daily for adults.	Individuals with kidney failure may be prone to developing magnesium toxicity. Taking large doses of laxatives or antacids that contain magnesium can be toxic.
Vitamin D	Vitamin D_3 is now known to be the more potent and active form (Armas, Hollis, and Heaney 2004).	Recommended daily intake from supplementation: 1000 IU (international units).	Vitamin D absorption is decreased by some medications, including steroids, orlistat (known as Xenical or alli for weight loss), and antiseizure (Dilantin) and cholesterol-lowering medications (Questran, Prevalite, LoCholest).

Calcium	Look for calcium in the form of calcium carbonate or calcium citrate.	Recommended daily intake (from food or supplementation): for adults under fifty: 1000 milligrams; for adults over fifty: 1200 milligrams.	Calcium may decrease levels of digoxin, a heart medication, and may interact with certain antibiotics (ciprofloxacin and tetracycline), thyroid medications, and Dilantin (an antiseizure medication).
B Vitamins	Take a B-complex vitamin. The B vitamins should be taken together to avoid, for example, intake of folic acid masking symptoms of B_{12} deficiency.	Recommended daily dosages in the B-complex vitamin (Institute of Medicine 1998): Folic acid: 1000 micrograms; B_{12}: 2.4 micrograms; B_6: 1.3 milligrams for men and women under the age of fifty, 1.5 milligrams for women over fifty, and 1.7 milligrams for men over fifty; thiamine (B_1): 1–2 milligrams; niacin (B_3): 15 milligrams. (Dosages to treat specific medical conditions—such as high cholesterol—should be recommended by your health care provider.)	High levels of folic acid may induce seizures in patients taking seizure medications. Taking large amounts of niacin may increase the risk of abnormal rhythms of the heart, can interfere with blood sugar control in diabetics, and may worsen gallbladder disease. Niacin is also not recommended for those with ulcers, liver disease, or severe low blood pressure.

Principle Five: Eat When You Are Hungry

This may be the most difficult of the five principles to follow. If you have BED or CO, you may be so used to feeding your emotional hunger that you're out of touch with the sensations of physical hunger. To learn this principle, you need to understand your hunger again.

WHY DON'T YOU FEEL HUNGRY NOW?

You may be someone who can go all day without eating and not feel any the worse for wear. Or you may find yourself feeling ravenous at the end of the day, which then leads you to binge. In order to get in touch with your hunger, you'll have to feed your body regularly for at least a month. This means eating three meals and a snack or two on a daily basis. Yes, this may mean you'll have to eat when you don't feel hungry. Your body may have adapted to the feast and famine cycle of BED/CO by shutting down your natural hunger cues. Eating regularly for a month will help these natural cues to return.

WHAT DOES NORMAL HUNGER FEEL LIKE?

"Normal" hunger refers to how you feel three to four hours after eating a regular, balanced meal. If you only ever feast or fast, or if you graze all day, never allowing your body to get hungry, you may not know what normal hunger and fullness feel like. Instead, you may only be familiar with extreme hunger and fullness. In reality, hunger is experienced on a sliding scale. Normally you should eat a meal at about a level two or three.

Hunger level 1: You may experience a little rumbling in your stomach.

Hunger level 2: Your stomach rumbling may increase. You may feel a mild burning sensation in your stomach.

Hunger level 3: You may have a slight headache.

Hunger level 4: You may sense an empty feeling in the pit of your stomach. You may start to think about eating. You may feel tired or agitated.

Hunger level 5: You may feel lightheaded or dizzy. You may be cranky and snap at people around you.

HOW DO YOU KNOW WHEN YOU'RE FULL?

The same level system can be applied to fullness. However, just as in the case of hunger, your current eating habits may be preventing you from recognizing when you are normally full or at a level three. Frequent bingeing may have stretched your stomach to the point that you can overfill it without receiving the normal body cues that you've gone too far.

Fullness level 1: Your hunger sensations begin to abate; you are still enjoying your meal.

Fullness level 2: If you were to stop eating, you'd feel satisfied but could still eat a little more.

Fullness level 3: You are comfortably full, satiated.

Fullness level 4: You're beginning to feel uncomfortably full.

Fullness level 5: You feel much too full; you can't stuff any more down; you feel sick or have stomach pain.

HOW CAN YOU TRUST YOUR HUNGER?

One reason you may be out of touch with your natural hunger cues, making it difficult to trust them, is that you're not eating regularly. Another reason may be that you're eating foods high in processed sugar and flour—cookies, cakes, candies, even fruit juice, bagels, and some other breads—foods that spike your blood sugar only to have it quickly dip to a very low level, triggering your hunger. (Foods that produce this effect are referred to as having a *high glycemic load*.)

Learning to listen to your body will, over time, enable you to trust your hunger. For example, under stress you may feel hungry for a chocolate bar. If you aren't sure you can trust this hunger, drink a glass of water first. If you decide to eat the chocolate, pay attention to your body's cues and notice when you feel hungry again. If you still feel hungry or if you become hungry within an hour of eating the chocolate, your body is telling you it needs something more substantial. If it is not a regular mealtime, eat a balanced snack that includes protein, healthy carbohydrates, and a bit of healthy fat (for example, an apple with peanut butter), then check in with your body again. Through this process, you'll learn what nourishes your body and what doesn't.

Assessing Your Hunger

As you sit down to your next meal, ask yourself:

1. Are you hungry? (Use the levels above to describe your hunger.) Level of hunger (from zero to five)

   _____

2. What are you feeling emotionally? (Bored, lonely, sad, happy, tired, and so on.)

   _____

3. If you aren't hungry, what does your body need at this moment? If you're tired, but it's not your usual bedtime, you may not have thought of just going to bed. If you're feeling an emotion strongly, consider whether it may be interfering with your hunger cues. If so, take a moment to describe how you're feeling below and then repeat this exercise. What you are feeling and how does this affect your ability to sense your hunger?

   _____

   _____

   _____

Remember: Healthy digestive function requires regular meals and snacks. It is best to eat before you feel as if you're starving and to stop eating when moderately full.

SUMMARY

It is difficult for anyone, including professionals, to interpret the many conflicting scientific recommendations about how and what to eat. Thus, instead of following a rigid nutrition plan, improve your eating habits by adopting the five principles described in this chapter little by little.

CHAPTER 4

Nourishing Your Body

written with Alicia Trocker, MS, RD

Transforming all of the conflicting information about nutrition into something resembling a healthy eating plan can be a daunting task. Sticking to it can be even more challenging. In this chapter we'll discuss macronutrients, calories, and meal planning, as well as how to handle curveballs such as holidays and foods that may trigger overeating or bingeing. Hang in there—nutrition clarity is around the corner! And remember: changing the way you eat is a process not a contest. Don't try to change everything all at once, as you would do with a diet. Instead, identify small changes you can make and pick your battles—don't try to force yourself to do something you're not ready to do.

MACRONUTRIENTS

In the previous chapter, we discussed how nutritional supplements can help provide your body with the healthy *micronutrients* (vitamins and minerals) it needs. Now, let's turn to *macronutrients* (the large units of nutrition): protein, carbohydrates, and fat. Macronutrients are what your body uses as fuel. Carbohydrates are the fastest and most readily available source of energy; when your body has used up all available carbohydrates, it then turns to protein and fat. When you overeat—even on healthy foods—the body stores extra food as fat.

Protein

Protein is needed for tissue repair, building muscle, immune function, growth, and making hormones and enzymes for digestion. When necessary, protein can also be broken down into energy. Protein is made of amino acids, most of which are essential—that is, we must get them from our diet as our bodies can't make them.

Get your protein from a variety of sources as each type of protein also offers other nutrients. For example, eggs are not just a source of protein, but also of vitamin A; milk contains both protein and calcium. Eat higher fat proteins in smaller amounts.

Sources of Protein

Lean	Medium Fat	High Fat
Fish	Lean beef	Peanut butter
Skinless chicken breast	Pork	Other nut butters
Egg whites	Eggs	Nuts
Nonfat plain yogurt	Low-fat cheese	Seeds
Nonfat (skim) or 1-percent milk	Salmon	High-fat meats such as salami, bacon, sausage, and fatty cuts of beef
Low-fat ricotta cheese	Low-fat milk (2 percent)	
Beans		Whole milk
Lentils		
Peas		

Carbohydrates

Carbohydrates are the body's main source of fuel or energy. Rich in B vitamins and minerals, carbohydrates help support the nervous system and build strong bones. Eating carbohydrates also increases the production of serotonin, a calming brain chemical.

Carbohydrates are categorized in terms of both their rating in the *glycemic index* and their *glycemic load*. The glycemic index ranks carbohydrates on a scale from one to a hundred based on the degree they increase blood sugar after eating. The glycemic load is a clarification of the glycemic index that takes into account the type and amount of carbohydrates you eat. For example, an apple has a lower glycemic load than a glass of apple juice. The glycemic load is thus a more accurate representation of the overall effect of the food on the body.

Carbohydrates that contain more fiber and less sugar take longer to be digested and have a lower glycemic load, providing energy over a longer period of time. These foods—also referred to as complex carbohydrates—include fruits, vegetables, and whole grains. On the other hand, simple carbohydrates—usually carbohydrates that have been processed or refined, such as white rice or white bread—have a higher glycemic load. Eating these foods will trigger a spike in blood sugar and the release of insulin.

Insulin then lowers blood sugar (which is why you can feel hungry shortly after eating a donut); insulin may also trigger the body to store unused energy (calories) as fat.

Some foods have a higher glycemic index rating but a lower glycemic load—for example, most fruits and beans. This is because you'd have to eat a lot of these foods for them to have a significant effect on blood sugar and insulin release. Foods that are slow to leave the stomach because they are high in fiber, have some acidity, or contain some fat tend to have a lower glycemic load. For example, carrots, although very sweet, have a low glycemic load due to their fiber. (Many books and websites offer more information on the glycemic load; see the resources section at the back of this book for more information on the glycemic load and other aspects of nutrition.)

Remember, even though processed or refined carbohydrates may be enriched, they've still lost most of their nutritional value. As an easy rule of thumb, foods that have a healthy (low) glycemic load usually require more chewing. For example, pasta cooked al dente (not quite soft) has a lower glycemic load than pasta cooked until soft.

Sources of Carbohydrates

Lower Glycemic Load (Complex Carbohydrates)	Higher Glycemic Load (Simple Carbohydrates)
Pumpernickel bread, buckwheat bread, cracked wheat kernel bread, rye bread	White bread, white wheat flour bread, white rice
Whole wheat, barley, millet, multigrain cereal	High-sugar cereals, donuts, pastries
Plain baked sweet potato/yam	Cookies, cakes, candies, pies
Plain microwave popcorn	Dried fruit
Fruits and non-starchy vegetables	Sodas
Legumes*: beans, lentils, peas	Bagels
Corn tortilla	

Foster-Powell, Holt, and Brand-Miller 2002

* Note that legumes are a source of both carbohydrates and protein.

Fats

Fats are a source of stored energy and contain essential fatty acids. As well, certain vitamins—A, D, E, and K—cannot be absorbed unless there is fat in the diet. Fats help maintain healthy skin and hair, promote healthy cell function, aid the production of sex hormones (estrogen, progesterone, and testosterone), and cushion our internal organs. Fats are classified as saturated, monounsaturated, or polyunsaturated. (Trans fats, discussed in the previous chapter, should be avoided if possible.)

Sources of Fats

Healthy Fats	Fats to Eat in Moderation	Fats to Avoid
Monounsaturated fats:	*Polyunsaturated fats:*	*Trans fats:*
Nut oils	Grapeseed oil	Microwave and theater popcorn
Olive oil	Safflower oil	Fried fast food
Canola oil	Sunflower oil	Many cookies
Flaxseeds	Soybean oil	Chips
Avocados	Sesame oil	Margarine
Walnuts	*Saturated fats:* Organic, unsalted butter	Many cakes and pies
	Coconut oil	

DON'T DEPRIVE YOURSELF, REWARD YOUR BODY WITH NOURISHMENT!

Don't deprive yourself. If you choose to eat higher-fat proteins, carbohydrates that have a higher glycemic load, or saturated fats (such as butter), just eat less of these in your overall diet than you do of the healthier versions of these foods. Focus on eating to nourish your body, rather than eating to lose weight.

CALORIES

Although calories are simply units that measure the energy available to you in the food you eat, in our fat-phobic, diet-crazy world just the word "calorie" has a lot of baggage associated with it. Rather than focus on calories, use one of the two following methods to determine how much you should eat.

Method 1: Eat Proportionally

For lunch and dinner, fill half of your plate with vegetables (for example, with salad), a quarter of your plate with a protein-rich food, and a quarter of your plate with other carbohydrates. If you are consuming smaller portions than usual, it can be helpful to eat clockwise—this way you'll get some of your favorite items throughout the meal. For breakfast, you still want to eat protein, a small amount of fat, and some carbohydrates. For example, you might eat steel-cut oatmeal with yogurt and fresh or frozen berries; or you might eat an egg or two (cooked in olive oil) with fresh vegetables and a slice of toast.

Method 2: Let Your Body Guide You

Let your body tell you whether you're eating enough or not. After you've followed some of the suggestions in the next section for changing how and what you eat, check how hungry you feel an hour after eating. If your hunger level is beyond level 2 only an hour after eating, you either haven't eaten enough food or what you ate didn't stay in your system long enough. Use your body's natural cues to fine-tune your eating habits, varying your meal choices to see which food combinations satisfy you longest. For example, if you are hungry soon after eating oatmeal with fruit, milk, and a half-teaspoon of butter, try replacing the butter with chopped nuts. If you're hungry soon after eating vegetable lasagna and a salad, try adding grilled chicken or beans to the lasagna or salad.

MENU PLANNING

Planning meals can be a challenge when you're changing how you eat. However, you already have some new tools to help you do so, the most important of which are your body's wisdom and its hunger/fullness levels. In a moment, we'll discuss some basic guidelines for planning what to eat; there are three steps to this process. But how will you know if your meal plan is working?

Review the following list of positive indicators daily, comparing them with how your body actually feels, then journal about your results on a weekly basis—this will help you collect important information about what works and doesn't work:

* Your desire to binge is reduced or eliminated

* Your food cravings go away

* You feel more energetic, better able to think clearly, less irritable

* You start to feel hungry at mealtimes

* You have normal digestion: no constipation, headaches, bloating, sluggishness, or gas

* You will be in the middle of your hunger level (about a level 3) before meals

Step 1: The Basics

Before you do anything else to your diet, see if you follow these guidelines for a week:

* Schedule a specific time for each meal and try to eat at the same time each day

* Eat three meals every day

* Eat two snacks a day

* Include all three macronutrients in each meal and snack: protein, fat, and carbohydrates

    *   Drink eight to ten glasses of water a day

    *   Move your body at least once a day, even if it's only for five minutes

Record your progress below. Mark each box where you were able to meet your goal. (You may want to copy this chart first to track your progress for even longer.)

GOAL	Monday	Tuesday	Wednesday	Thursday	Friday	Saturday	Sunday
Ate on schedule							
Ate three meals							
Ate two snacks							
Included protein, fat, and carbs at each meal/snack							
Drank 8–10 glasses of water							
Physical activity for at least five minutes							

Good job! Now on to step two.

Step 2: Changing How and What You Eat

For step two, continue what you learned in step one and add to it by choosing meals that will nourish your body, mind, and spirit (a list of meal ideas follows). Then, record how eating these meals makes you feel. From the following list select three meals and two snacks. Mix it up. The list also includes suggestions for drinks and sweeteners. Diet drinks are not a healthy alternative to drinks with high fructose corn syrup. Heavy use of diet sweeteners such as aspartame has been linked to seizures and other health risks, including cancer (Huff and LaDou 2007). Desserts are not included on the list because they are trigger foods for many people with BED/CO. (We'll discuss trigger foods further in the Special Topics section at the end of the chapter.)

    The following meal suggestions are not meant to be a diet plan. If you have a medical condition, such as high cholesterol or diabetes, that requires a special diet, you should discuss your meal plan with your health care provider or a registered dietician. Try to make healthy choices for fats, proteins, and carbohydrates the majority of the time. For meals including milk, you may want to use lower fat milk (nonfat or 1 percent), as milk is high in saturated fat.

In general, look for ways to add herbs—particularly fresh herbs—and spices to your cooking. Herbs and spices have their own healing power. For example, rosemary promotes digestion, sage helps prevent colds and sore throats, and basil soothes nerves and helps alleviate depression. In addition, garlic helps lower blood pressure and increases our ability to fight off colds and infections, turmeric has anticancer properties, and ginger is an anti-inflammatory. Besides that, they make meals flavorful!

Breakfast	Hot cereal* (oatmeal or millet) with nonfat or 1-percent milk** and blueberries or other fruit; for more protein, add nuts or seeds
	Whole wheat toast, eggs (poached or cooked with olive oil spray), and fruit; add veggies to your eggs for extra nutrients
	Breakfast burrito: eggs, salsa, and black beans wrapped in a corn tortilla with a sprinkle of cheese; orange slices
	Cold cereal (Kashi or Cheerios) with nonfat or 1-percent milk, and fruit; for more protein, add nuts or seeds
	Veggie omelet: combine whole eggs with egg whites, then add salsa or veggies like spinach, bell peppers, onions, mushrooms
	Toast with peanut butter and a smoothie***
	Multigrain pancakes or french toast with turkey sausage and fresh fruit
Lunch	Turkey chili with cornbread and veggie salad (cucumber, tomatoes, bell peppers)
	Salad of chopped vegetables, dark greens, and turkey, fish, or chicken, dressed with olive oil and balsamic vinegar, plus a slice of whole grain bread
	Broth-based soup (add extra vegetables) and a salad or sandwich; for something sweet, add fruit
	Tuna fish sandwich with salad made from chopped cucumbers, tomatoes, red onions, and carrots
	Chicken pasta salad: macaroni pasta, chopped chicken, celery, onions, and carrots (or your favorite veggies), dressed with olive oil and balsamic vinegar instead of mayo
	Bean soup and tortilla or pita chips, plus apple and string cheese
	Fajitas with corn or whole wheat tortillas and salad; fajitas can be vegetarian or made with your favorite lean meat

Dinner	Moo shu vegetable or moo shu chicken, stir-fried veggies, and brown rice
	Large greek salad: feta cheese, olives, cucumbers, plus hummus and pita bread.
	Grilled salmon, small green salad, rice pilaf, green beans or squash or other non-starchy vegetable
	Vegetable lasagna, mixed greens salad with sliced pears and walnuts; for more protein, add kidney or garbanzo beans to the salad
	Soft chicken taco, cup of tortilla soup, and salad
	Turkey, baked yam, steamed cauliflower or brussels sprouts or broccoli, plus a small tossed salad with tomatoes
	Whole-grain pasta**** with garlic marinara sauce (add chopped veggies to sauce when cooking) and chicken or shrimp, plus salad caprese: sliced tomatoes, fresh basil leaves, and thinly sliced mozzarella drizzled with one teaspoon each of olive oil and balsamic vinegar
Snacks	10–15 walnuts, mixed nuts, or almonds combined with a tablespoon of raisins or cranberries, or your favorite dried fruit
	Apple slices with almond or peanut butter
	Pear slices with cheddar cheese
	Celery sticks or baby carrots with hummus or bean dip
	Whole-grain crackers and cheese
	Nonfat plain or lemon yogurt with 6–10 nuts and chopped fruit
	Low-fat cottage cheese with fresh fruit
Drinks	Water; add lemon, lime, cucumber, or basil leaves
	Iced or hot tea, especially green, white, or oolong tea
	Nonfat or 1-percent milk
	Vegetable juice such as V-8 or Bloody Mary mix (virgin); use low sodium V-8 if you have high blood pressure
	Fruit juice; limit to one cup a day
	Mix sparkling water or club soda with a quarter- to a half-cup of fruit juice
Sweeteners *****	Stevia
	Dark maple syrup (grade C)
	Honey
	Agave

* If you don't have one minute in your day to cook oatmeal, look for Amy's brand frozen whole-grain cereals that can be heated in the microwave.

** You can substitute soy or almond milk in any of the meals that include milk.

*** Smoothie: blend one cup of frozen berries, a half-cup of low-fat milk, 5–6 ice cubes, and half a container of nonfat yogurt (unflavored) in an electric blender; for a sweeter taste, add stevia or a quarter of a ripe banana; for more nutrients, add three tablespoons of wheat germ or one scoop of whey protein powder.

**** You can purchase whole-grain pasta from many grocery or whole food stores.

*****For more information on healthy sweeteners see *Healing Foods for Dummies* (Siple 1999).

Step 3: Develop Your Individual Meal Plan

For step three, first write up your meal plan for the next week—sit down and work on this before your work week begins. Ready, set, get started…

Menu Plan

	Breakfast	Lunch	Dinner	Snack 1	Snack 2
Monday					
Tuesday					
Wednesday					
Thursday					
Friday					
Saturday					
Sunday					

Next, make copies of the following meal diary to use each day. Every day, record your level of hunger, any emotions you're feeling around a meal or during the day, what food you actually eat, and your fullness level after eating.

Meal Diary

Date: _____

	Hunger Level (0–5)	Emotions	Food Eaten	Fullness Level (0–5)
Breakfast				
Lunch				
Dinner				
Snack 1				
Snack 2				

Continue to track what you eat, planning your menu on the same day each week. This practice will help you be accountable to yourself. Thus, every week you will record what you plan to eat and then what you actually ate, along with your hunger and fullness levels and the emotions you experienced. Every week you will also plan the next week's menus. (See the resources section at the back of this book for websites about nutrition and meal planning; there are many meal-planning software programs available as well.)

SPECIAL TOPICS

Let's turn now to some of the particular challenges you may face while trying to improve your nutritional status.

Metabolic Rate

You may feel that you have a lower metabolism than other people and therefore need to eat less in order not to gain weight. If you are concerned your metabolism is lower than normal, many fitness clubs offer a test that will tell you what your metabolic rate is and the resultant number of calories you need to eat to maintain your weight. Metabolism is affected by age, sex (men have faster metabolisms), and medical conditions (underactive thyroid).

Even if your metabolic rate is low, there are things you can do to increase it. For example, exercise and weight training can both build lean muscle, making you more efficient at burning fat. And aerobic exercise done in the morning can boost your metabolism for most of the day, burning calories even when you are no longer exercising. However, do not skip meals, especially breakfast. Eating early and frequently throughout the day stimulates your body's "engine" to burn calories. In the beginning, as your body adjusts to eating regularly, you may experience a slight weight gain. This is because your body is used to holding onto the calories it gets when you feast in order to prepare for the fast it knows is coming. With time, eating regularly will boost your metabolism and your weight will decrease to a healthy level.

Trigger Foods

Trigger foods are foods you just can't resist—when you start eating them, you often can't stop. In the following exercise, note any foods that trigger you to overeat or binge.

Your Trigger Foods

List below any foods you tend to binge on or often find yourself overeating. Remember: these are the foods that you can't resist if you have them in the house. A few of the more common ones have already been put on the list to get you started:

Ice cream

Cookies

Chips

Chocolate, chocolate candies, or chocolate anything

_____

_____

_____

Now, write down the feelings you experience before and after eating a trigger food:

Before eating _____

I feel _____

_____

After eating _____

I feel _____

_____

You may find that particular foods have a heavy-duty emotional charge for you. If you think it would be useful, analyze for yourself why in your journal. For example, why do you like chocolate so much?

Biological reasons (such as the need for feel-good brain chemicals like serotonin) often draw us to certain foods. However, if you follow the suggestions in this chapter, your excessive desire for trigger foods will subside over time. In the meantime:

* Always have your trigger food available to you (in a small quantity). For example, if ice cream is your trigger food, purchase a four-ounce container of your favorite ice cream and keep it in your freezer.

* When you decide to eat a trigger food, eat it after a meal or snack, not in place of a meal or snack.

* When you are eating your trigger food, put all of your attention and focus on how it tastes, describing it to yourself in detail; enjoy the physical sensation of eating it. For example: *I love the creamy-sweet flavor of peppermint ice cream with its crunchy bits of candy. It feels smooth and yet there are little surprises of happiness when I bite into the candy bits.*

* Whatever you do, whatever you eat, do not judge yourself or beat yourself up. If you find yourself starting to do this, get up and distract yourself—take a walk, watch TV, make a phone call. Break the cycle of negative self-talk and you will break the bond between you and your trigger foods.

Holidays

How can you stay on a healthy eating plan during the holidays? In the beginning it will be very difficult. Here are some tips to help you survive holidays:

* Don't ever try to diet during the holidays.

* Enjoy eating what you want but be careful of overeating.

* Make the healthiest choices possible given the circumstances.

* Watch how much alcohol you drink, both because alcohol can make it difficult to make wise decisions and because alcoholic drinks can contain a high number of calories.

* Don't skip meals to compensate for how much you've previously eaten. This will just make it more likely that you'll overeat or binge at the next meal.

* Enjoy being with friends and family. Focus more on this and less on the food.

SUMMARY

Whether it's modifying how and what you eat, starting to exercise, or stopping smoking, changing your behavior is never easy. Permanent change takes time. If you've been in the habit of dramatically modifying your eating habits while on a diet, you may have a skewed perspective of how much time these kinds of changes should take. Changes in your eating habits should be accomplished over a period of months and years, not weeks. Making small changes that you can sustain is more effective in the longterm than making sweeping changes—as you do on short-term diets—that you can't. In this journey, it's much better to be the tortoise than the hare.

PART 2

Healing the Mind

CHAPTER 5

Overview of Traditional Approaches to BED/CO

Various conventional approaches have been used to treat BED/CO, including cognitive behavioral therapy (CBT), dialectical behavior therapy (DBT), interpersonal psychotherapy (IPT), and medications, in addition to the dietary recommendations and exercise discussed in previous chapters. This chapter offers an overview of the most common forms of therapy and medication that have been found effective in decreasing unhealthy behaviors, addressing body dissatisfaction, and reducing depression in individuals with BED/CO.

The first goal of therapy should be interrupting any current unhealthy behaviors, such as bingeing or overeating. The majority of people with BED have very chaotic eating patterns: they eat more, both at meals and during binges, than people who are obese but don't have BED (Goldfein et al. 1993); they tend to engage in weight cycling, or yo-yo dieting (Yanovski 1993); they eat over longer periods of time; and finally, they are unable to regulate their eating behavior both during and between binge episodes (Guss et al. 1994).

Therapy should also help you both identify and heal the root causes of your eating disorder. This may require changing how you feel about your body. Although you may not desire the extreme skinniness that someone with anorexia nervosa tries to achieve, if you have BED/CO you're likely to suffer from poor body image, experiencing strong feelings of dissatisfaction with your body.

If you suffer from depression and/or anxiety—or if you've been diagnosed with a personality disorder that is affecting your relationships with your family or friends—therapy can help. (We'll discuss this further in chapter 9.) Both BED and CO can increase symptoms of depression—and depression can increase your weight and bingeing (Stunkard, Fernstrom et al. 1990). Indeed, you can gain as much as seventeen pounds during an episode of depression (Weissenburger et al. 1986). Research has shown that the severity of depression in individuals with BED is directly related to the frequency of their binges (Marcus et al. 1990).

COGNITIVE BEHAVIORAL THERAPY (CBT)

Cognitive behavioral therapy (CBT) is based on the idea that our feelings and behaviors are caused by what we think rather than by things outside of ourselves, such as other people, situations, and events. A very common form of therapy, CBT is meant to be brief. During a limited period of time, clients learn to manage their perceptions of and reactions to the problems in their lives. For example, a common scenario in my office is a patient who is convinced that her father—or some other person in her life—is the cause of all of her problems, including her eating disorder. This patient therefore has two problems: an unhealthy or unfulfilling relationship with her father and her reaction to this relationship. In CBT, clients are encouraged to check their perceptions of a situation by asking questions such as, "How do I know that what I believe is really what is occurring?" and "What are my perceptions and what are the facts?" CBT is based on learning to recognize the facts of a situation; these facts are then used to challenge perceptions and identify inaccurate assumptions or conclusions.

Cognitive Behavioral Therapy Research

In treating BED and CO, the focus of CBT is on moderation—i.e., on reducing extreme behaviors of *restricting* (fasting or not eating regularly) or overeating. Several research studies support the use of CBT in treating BED and CO. CBT has been shown to reduce bingeing for up to four months after the end of treatment (Brownley et al. 2007). Pairing CBT with hypnosis is an effective treatment combination, particularly for treating obesity (Kirsch, Montgomery, and Sapirstein 1995). Finally, CBT is more effective in treating BED/CO when treatment is over a longer period of time (for example, twenty-two sessions in twenty-four weeks) (Marcus 1997).

Cognitive Behavioral Therapy and BED/CO

If you choose to see a therapist who uses CBT, you will most likely work through three stages of CBT: The first eight sessions will focus on skills that will both help you eat regular meals on a daily basis and decrease binge behaviors. The next eight sessions will address decreasing food intake without restricting what you eat and will challenge the thoughts and beliefs that perpetuate your eating disorder. The final six sessions will be devoted to the maintenance of the progress you've made and the prevention of relapses. While you may lose weight during treatment with CBT, the primary goal is not weight loss. Indeed, weight loss issues should be handled separately, and only after the primary goals have been accomplished: bingeing is reduced, eating is more normal and less chaotic, and unhealthy beliefs have been addressed.

CBT can also help address the enormous shame you may feel about your binge eating or compulsive overeating. This experience of shame can include feelings of helplessness, inferiority, anger, and fear of being judged by others. Shame can come from your own feelings about your body or from your perceptions or experiences of being judged by others because of your size (Gilbert, Pehl, and Allan 1994). It is important to address this shame as it may exacerbate or perpetuate depression, creating a vicious cycle in which shame and depression drive the unhealthy behaviors associated with BED/CO (Andrews 1995).

If you are interested in CBT, you can contact the National Association of Cognitive-Behavioral Therapists to find a certified therapist (see the resources section for more information). However, not all CBT therapists will have experience treating BED or CO; interview therapists you're considering to ascertain their level of experience with the issues you want to address.

DIALECTICAL BEHAVIOR THERAPY (DBT)

Initially, dialectical behavior therapy (DBT) was used to treat clients suffering from severe depression, self-destructive behavior, and borderline personality disorder (more on this in chapter 11). Later, DBT came to be used to treat many other difficult to treat conditions, including eating disorders. The DBT concepts and exercises in this section have been adapted from Marsha Linehan's *Skills Training Manual for Treating Borderline Personality Disorder* (1993) with permission from The Guilford Press.

A combination of cognitive behavioral therapy and Buddhist concepts of mindfulness, DBT involves practice exercises designed to teach clients to better tolerate emotional distress, improve their ability to form healthy relationships, and cope with their emotions without being dominated or controlled by them. The skills you learn from DBT can help you sort through conflicting emotions and tolerate situations that you cannot change.

DBT theory views pain as part of the human condition and distinct from suffering. Suffering is defined as nonacceptance of pain. For example, if you go through a divorce after twenty years of marriage, you will experience pain in the form of anger, sorrow, fear, and other emotions. Suffering comes about when, instead of accepting your feelings, you blame other people for how you feel, get stuck in feeling sorry for yourself, or distract yourself from your true emotions. DBT can help you if you want to move on and just don't know how.

Dialectical Behavior Therapy Research

One study found that 89 percent of individuals with BED who were taught DBT stopped bingeing; six months later, 56 percent still abstained from binge behaviors (Telch, Agras, and Linehan 2001). In another group of individuals with BED, DBT was found to be very successful in reducing binge behavior and moderately successful in decreasing mood disorder symptoms and suicidal and self-harm behavior (Chen et al. 2008). Presently no studies have examined the use of DBT with CO.

Dialectical Behavior Therapy and BED/CO

You can learn the basic principles of DBT from a therapist who uses DBT techniques or from a DBT group. However, with its emphasis on exercises and skills, in order to truly learn DBT, you must experience what happens when you use DBT in a distressing situation. To do so, DBT skills must be practiced daily and integrated into your life. DBT skills that I have found particularly helpful in my work with BED and CO are its mindfulness skills and skills that help you tolerate distress.

DBT MINDFULNESS SKILLS

The mindfulness skills of DBT come from the Buddhist tradition (for more information, see, for example, Thich Nhat Hahn's *The Miracle of Mindfulness*). When you are mindful, you observe and describe what you are experiencing, even when the experience is painful. Mindfulness allows you to just "sit" with your experience—to participate in what you are feeling and change your reactions to harmful situations as a result. One of the most important elements of mindfulness is learning not to judge your emotions, the emotions of others, or your situation. Such judgments are common—for example, we often describe things as good or bad. When you separate the facts from your emotions, you can focus on situations without labeling them. This will help you determine what is helpful and what is not; from there, you can do whatever will work best in the situation.

Mindfulness

1. Write down a recent situation that you found painful or upsetting: (Example: *I was fired from my job.*)

    _____

    _____

    _____

2. Describe how you felt about what happened: (Example: *I was extremely angry—I'd worked my butt off at that job. I was also afraid because I don't have a lot of savings and wasn't sure I'd be able to pay my bills. I also wondered if I was fired because I'm overweight.*)

    _____

    _____

    _____

3. List your thoughts about the situation: (Example: *My boss was out to get me. As soon as I took the job, he and I didn't get along. I think he turned my coworkers against me.*)

    _____

    _____

    _____

4. Next, fully describe the emotions you listed in response to question number 2 as well as any physical sensations you remember: (Example: *I felt my face flush and my heart race. My whole body was shaking with anger. Later, fear just took me over. I felt panicky and jittery. I felt like I was going to be sick.*)

_____

_____

_____

5. See if you can unhook your feelings, opinions, and judgments from the facts: (The facts are the who, what, when, and where of the situation.)

Facts	Judgments	Opinions
Example: _Yesterday my boss fired me._	_My boss is a jerk._	_I wasn't treated fairly._

Review the chart above. If you have statements in the facts column that include judgments or emotions, rewrite them to focus just on the facts. Remember: a fact is something that can objectively be shown to be true; facts are the circumstances of an event or situation, not interpretations of it.

6. Next, think about ways to resolve your situation, if possible. If you can't completely resolve it, think of actions you can take to make things better for yourself—to reduce the emotional damage and allow you to move forward. Avoid actions that originate in spite or other emotions. Act from reality, not from what you wish would have happened. Focus on the big picture—not just on what is happening right now but on your deeper goals. Try not to act from self-righteousness or anger, as this will hurt you more than it will hurt others you may want revenge on.

    List at least five things you could do that would help you resolve the situation: (Example: _I will get listed with a temp agency. I will make a budget and find ways to decrease spending until I find another job. I will contact my networking group and ask them for leads for new jobs._)

_____

_____

_____

7. Make a list of obstacles that may hinder you in accomplishing your five goals. Next to each obstacle, write at least one action you can take to minimize or eliminate it:

Obstacle	Corrective Action
Example: *Fear of what other people will think about me because of being fired.*	*I will discuss with my therapist how to address my fear and develop a plan for responding to questions from prospective employers.*

SKILLS THAT HELP YOU TOLERATE DISTRESS

We experience distress when things don't go our way, situations are upsetting but cannot immediately be changed, and relationships don't meet our needs. Very sensitive individuals may feel things more strongly than others, taking offense even when no offense is meant. Because distress can be difficult to tolerate, you may have found yourself overeating, bingeing, drinking, or engaging in other unhealthy behaviors to get rid of unpleasant feelings.

There are four types of skills for improving distress tolerance: skills of distraction, self-soothing skills, skills for immediately improving the moment, and the pros and cons skill.

Skills of distraction. Distraction can put distance between a current situation and your feelings. Bingeing or overeating may have become an automatic response to certain stimuli (negative comments about your appearance, negative thoughts you have, stress, and so on). However, you can intentionally use distraction to interrupt the stimuli and emotionally charged thoughts that lead to these unhealthy behaviors. There are many different ways to distract yourself. Examples include taking a walk, calling a friend, taking three deep breaths, and reading.

One distraction skill that has been particularly helpful to many of my patients is the skill of *push away* or leaving a situation alone for a time. To do this, imagine yourself putting the problem into a lockbox and then storing that box on the top shelf of your closet until you are less emotional or have more support and are ready to take it out and deal with it.

Self-soothing skills. Self-soothing skills help you nurture and calm yourself. Many people with BED/CO either don't feel they deserve to be nurtured or expect someone else to do it for them. Learning to self-soothe is part of learning to love yourself and to accept that you deserve to be loved. The skills of self-soothing employ the five senses. For example, you might soothe yourself by taking a bubble bath, smelling a rose, listening to music, or noticing the beauty of nature.

Skills for immediately improving the moment. Various skills can help you immediately change things in the moment; these include prayer, relaxation, using your imagination (e.g., thinking of a beautiful beach you've visited), and finding meaning in your pain. These skills help you to immediately transform a negative situation into a more positive one through shifting your perceptions and physical responses and letting go. Because these skills tap into the mind-body connection, they allow you to transcend the tumult of thoughts and emotions you may be feeling. Thus, like the old commercial on television, one moment you may be cleaning up a messy spill in your kitchen with three kids hanging onto your leg and the dog barking, while the next you may be whisked away to a relaxing Calgon bubble bath on a beach in Bali (at least in your imagination).

Pros and cons skill. When you analyze your current situation for its pros and cons you discover all the different ways the situation does and doesn't serve you. This can help you become better aware of the benefits of tolerating your distress rather than continuing unhealthy ways of coping such as smoking cigarettes, bingeing, overeating, drinking, or engaging in other impulsive and hurtful behaviors.

An in-depth discussion of each of these skills is outside the scope of this book. However, the following exercises will give you a sense of the skills that my patients with BED/CO have found to be helpful.

Distress Tolerance

Describe a situation related to your BED/CO that you found difficult to deal with. For example, a holiday with your family when someone commented on your weight. You can choose a situation that no longer bothers you or one that still bothers you to this day:

_____

_____

_____

_____

What did you do at that time to cope or make yourself feel better? (Example: *I tried to tell myself that she hadn't meant to hurt me. When that didn't work, I went into the kitchen after everyone else had left and binged.*)

_____

_____

_____

_____

Circle skills on the following list that could have helped you in this particular situation. Remember, DBT skills are not meant to *solve* problems. They are meant to give you some distance from problems or situations and the ability to not act immediately when you are feeling emotional or when a situation is uncomfortable.

Skill list:

Go to a movie

Work on a crossword puzzle

Ride a bike

Talk to a friend; ask the friend for support

Pray

Read an inspirational book

Take a hot bath and put lavender lotion on your skin (lavender is stress reducing)

Listen to relaxing music

Get a massage

Meditate

Practice just sitting with your feelings without judging them

Imagine yourself in a relaxing place, such as at a beach or in the mountains

Take three deep breaths

_____

_____

_____

_____

In the next exercise, analyze the advantages and disadvantages of not acting from your emotions—i.e., learning to tolerate distress. Do this exercise with your BED/CO in mind. How would it affect your eating disorder if you stopped acting from emotions? What are the advantages and disadvantages of doing so? Finding pros for learning to tolerate distress is easy: if you were better at managing your emotions, you would stop bingeing, you would lose weight, your life would be improved. But you'd also give up certain things. For example, if you stopped using food to manage your distress, you'd no longer enjoy the instant gratification that comes with doing so. Ceasing your bingeing behaviors may also affect your relationships with your family. Do you get a lot of attention because of your eating disorder, even if it's negative attention? Dig deep for the next exercise. Be as honest as you can about how your eating disorder helps and hurts you.

Pros and Cons

The pros and cons of tolerating distress rather than acting from your emotions:

_____

_____

_____

_____

_____

_____

How will learning to tolerate your emotions and using DBT skills to deal with the crises in your life affect your BED/CO?

_____

_____

_____

_____

_____

_____

_____

These skills only work with practice. In the next exercise, record every time you practice a skill and whether the skill reduced your distress level. In the beginning, it may seem like the skills are not working. Believe me, they work. You just have to practice. The better you get at using these skills, the more likely they are to reduce your emotional distress.

Weekly Skills Practice

Use the descriptions of the different types of skills and the skill list from the preceding exercise to choose at least two skills to practice every day. Try to practice the same two skills for a week; for example, you might practice the skills of push away and soothing the five senses. Make a copy of the following skills chart so that you can use it next week, too, when you will practice another two skills daily.

See if you can identify at least five skills that are very effective for you. These should be skills that can be used in a variety of situations. Obviously, if you get upset at work you can't stop and take a hot bath. You'll need another skill to use until you can get home. Don't forget to try the mindfulness skills of observing and describing your emotions, being nonjudgmental, and sitting with your feelings.

Rate your level of distress using a scale of one to ten, with one being not upset at all (you're relaxed and calm) and ten being very upset (you want to explode). Rate your distress both before you use the skill and after; this will help you determine if the skill you used helped decrease your level of distress. Before you decide whether a skill is working or not, make sure you practice it a number of times. If you consistently find that a particular skill isn't helping you, try another. But make sure you give a skill at least a week before you give up on it.

The following is a sample weekly skills practice chart to help you get started.

	Skills to Practice This Week	Distress Rating Before Practicing Skill (0–10)	Distress Rating After Practicing Skill (0–10)	Situation	Comments
Monday	1. Distraction: walked around the mall once.	8	7	Urge to binge on popcorn at the movies.	I still binged This is not working for me!
	2. Self-soothing: listened to music.	9	5	Mom called and asked me how my diet was going.	Sometimes I just can't believe my mom. She's so thoughtless.
Tuesday	1. Distraction: called a friend to talk.	10	6	Doctor's visit; I got weighed.	I felt better after talking to Margie.
	2. Self-soothing: took a bath.	7	3	Tried on an old pair of jeans and couldn't get into them.	I wish I could get back to my old weight.

Wednesday	1. Distraction: went to a movie instead of going home to binge.	12+	9	Broke up with my girlfriend.	It helped to distract myself. When I got home, I also called a friend to talk.
	2. Pros and cons: wrote down pros and cons of the relationship.	9	2	Got a text message from ex-girlfriend's best friend.	I know she's calling to discuss the breakup and I'm not ready to do this.
Thursday	I didn't practice any skills today.	10		Ex-girlfriend called; we argued.	Life sucks!
Friday	1. Distraction: went to the gym.	9	7	Felt sad and angry after work when I had to go home alone.	I know I need to get my emotions and my eating under control.
	2. Self-soothing: sat in hot tub at gym.	5	3	Seeing all the buff people at the gym depressed me.	At least I worked out. I feel proud of myself.
Saturday	1. Distraction: watched TV.	9	6	My friend cancelled on me. We were supposed to have coffee together.	I can see that I need to keep doing stuff no matter how bad I feel. When I get out of the house I feel better.
	2. Self-soothing: went to the botanical gardens.	6	3		
Sunday	1. Distraction: push away.	8	3	Woke up worrying: will I ever have a family and someone who loves me?	I will focus on the now and on getting healthy first.
	2. Self-soothing: got a massage.	6	0	Got a text message from ex-girlfriend.	Brought up more feelings. Skills are helping a little.

	Skills to Practice This Week	Distress Rating Before Practicing Skill (0–10)	Distress Rating After Practicing Skill (0–10)	Situation	Comments
Monday					
Tuesday					
Wednesday					
Thursday					
Friday					
Saturday					
Sunday					

This is but a sampling of the skills you can learn from DBT; these skills can help put you in the driver's seat with your emotions, so that they no longer control you. If you want more support in using DBT skills than this, look for therapists who use DBT or a DBT group (see the resources section for more information); if you are currently in therapy, ask your therapist for a referral.

INTERPERSONAL PSYCHOTHERAPY (IPT)

Interpersonal psychotherapy (IPT) is a short-term, very structured type of therapy, originally developed for the treatment of depression. Since then it has been used to treat a number of other diagnoses, and has been shown to be effective in reducing the risk of relapse in eating disorders (Keel 2005). IPT is based on the theory that the interpersonal situations we experience in life can lead to the development of psychological problems in vulnerable individuals. Examples of interpersonal problems that this type of therapy addresses include: conflict with others (e.g., arguments with a spouse), grief, transitions (e.g., starting college, getting married or divorced), and lack of relationships and social support. The goal of IPT in treating BED/CO is to examine interpersonal problems and use any insights gained to change eating behaviors. Symptoms related to the eating disorder itself are not specifically addressed. For this reason, IPT is sometimes combined with CBT.

Interpersonal Therapy Research

Research has shown that IPT is as effective as CBT in treating binge eating disorder. A year after treatment, patients treated with IPT had reduced their number of binge days by 50 percent; those treated with CBT had reduced their binge days by 55 percent (Wilfley et al. 1993).

MEDICATIONS

Medications have been used in treating BED/CO to target mood disorders, weight loss, and eating behaviors.

Research on Medications for BED/CO

Several medications have shown promise in treating BED/CO. (I'll refer to these medications by their popular names rather than their generic names so they're easier to recognize.) Research has focused on three categories of medications in treating binge eating disorder and compulsive overeating: antiseizure medications, antidepressants, and anti-obesity agents.

ANTISEIZURE MEDICATIONS

Topamax is a medication used to treat seizure disorders and to stabilize the mood of patients with bipolar disorder. One study found that Topamax reduces bingeing behavior in obese individuals with BED; Topamax also lowers appetite—perhaps as a result, participants in this study lost weight (McElroy et al. 2007). The common side effects of Topamax include dizziness, insomnia, depression, nausea, difficulty with concentration, and attention and memory problems. The usual dosage range is 200 to 400 milligrams per day, divided into two doses.

ANTIDEPRESSANTS

Most of the antidepressants that have been tested in treating BED increase serotonin in the brain. For example, some research suggests Prozac and Zoloft may decrease bingeing behavior and help obese persons with BED to lose weight (Leombruni et al. 2008). However, other research found neither Prozac alone nor Prozac combined with CBT to be effective in treating BED (Grilo et al. 2005). Other medications in this category that reduce bingeing and body weight over the short term include Luvox and Celexa (Appolinario and McElroy 2004). In most studies, higher doses were used to treat binge eating disorder (60 milligrams) than were used to treat depression (20–40 milligrams). Short-term side effects of drugs in this category include nausea, diarrhea, headaches, and agitation; these side effects usually resolve after taking the medication for two to three weeks. Other common side effects that may occur after taking these medications for more than one month include insomnia, changes in sexual response (decrease in sex drive, delay in achieving orgasm), and—in some—weight gain. For this reason, further studies are needed to see if the initial weight loss patients experience is greater than the potential weight gain associated with taking the medications long term.

ANTI-OBESITY AGENTS

Of the anti-obesity agents, Meridia is the most well-studied in treating binge eating disorder and obesity. Preliminary evidence supports the use of Meridia (15 milligrams daily) to reduce binge frequency, enhance weight loss (approximately nine pounds), decrease body mass index, and reduce disordered eating behaviors (Milano et al. 2005; Wilfley et al. 2008). Research found it did not affect quality of life measures such as vitality, general health, or mental health more than a placebo (Wilfley et al. 2008). Side effects of Meridia include dry mouth, headache, constipation, insomnia, and dizziness.

SUMMARY

Many types of therapy and medication can improve your chances of long-term recovery. If you still think you can do it on your own and don't want to seek outside help or support, ask yourself how long you've been going it alone. Use the DBT skill of analyzing pros and cons to see whether going it alone has primarily helped you or held you back. If you're doing great on your own, stick with it. If, on the other hand, you're ready for outside help and support, use the information in this chapter to become a more educated consumer.

CHAPTER 6

What's Food Got to Do with BED/CO?

You may have wondered why, despite many attempts on your part, it's so difficult to stop bingeing or compulsive overeating. This is because behaviors, emotions, core beliefs, body sensations, and the deeper urges of the soul or spirit are all connected. (For "soul" or "spirit," substitute whatever word fits for you: higher power, bliss, healthy self, and so on.) This chapter will focus on the role of these interconnections in BED/CO.

What I've learned from my years of working with patients with BED/CO is that food's role in these disorders is actually very small. Many of my patients who binge admit that they don't even really taste the food they're eating. Food provides them with relief from emotions, comfort or a feeling of being nurtured, and an opportunity to escape from life's doldrums and pains. So, if BED and CO aren't about food, what *are* they about? The following diagram shows the different elements you'll need to deal with as you move toward recovery from BED/CO. Each level here drives the next; the arrows represent the order most people progress through these levels during the process of recovery.

Finding Your Anchor: The Process of Recovery

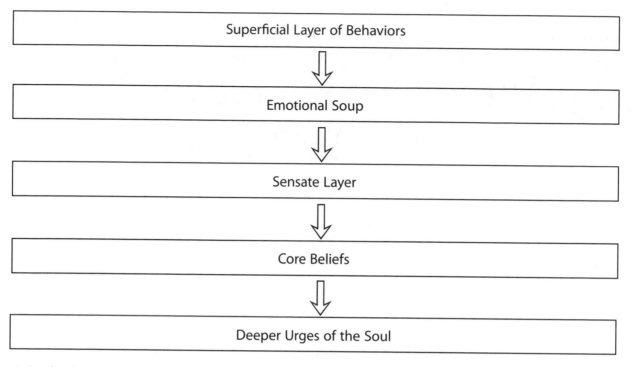

© Carolyn Ross, 2005

When you don't address and transform all of these levels, behaviors will return. Maybe you've already found this to be true. Ultimately, the healing process is about getting back to your true self, the self that expresses the deeper urges of your soul. Your soul self is the anchor that sustains you in recovery even when things get tough. Let's turn now to exploring each level and the healing it requires.

THE SUPERFICIAL LAYER OF BEHAVIORS

It's important to hold yourself accountable for your behaviors. You make choices every day about what you eat, whether to binge or overeat, whether to hoard or sneak food, whether or not to exercise, and how you treat your body in general. These behaviors may help you cope with problems in your life—stress, difficult relationships, emotional upsets, and so on. You may also employ other behaviors unrelated to eating for the same reasons. For example, you may drink too much, abuse sex, or shop compulsively as a way to cope when you're stressed out.

All of these behaviors have secondary consequences. One consequence of bingeing and compulsive shopping is greater financial stress. Even if you have parents or a spouse who supports you and pays your bills, running up huge credit card bills can cause conflict and resentment in your relationship. Use the following exercise to come clean about all of the ways your actions disrupt your life, cause you—and others—pain, affect your health and well-being, and create distance between you and those you care about. This exercise will be seen by you and only you, so don't hold back. And don't worry about any feelings of shame or guilt right now; we'll be working on emotions in the next section.

The Consequences of Your Behaviors

Mark the behaviors below that apply to you and that you are ready to hold yourself accountable for; if behaviors specifically related to your BED/CO are not on the list, write them in below:

Hiding food so people won't see you eat

Eating very little when you're at a meal with other people so they won't judge you

Lying about what you've eaten when asked

Bingeing or overeating at night when no one's awake

Hoarding food

Stealing food

Bingeing on food in the grocery store that you don't pay for

Running up credit card debt because of bingeing or overeating

_____

_____

_____

Next, list disruptive or unhealthy behaviors that aren't specifically related to your BED/CO but that you're ready to hold yourself accountable for:

Abusing alcohol

Abusing drugs

Using sex in unhealthy ways

Being a workaholic

Being a compulsive shopper (if so, what is your current level of debt?)

_____

_____

_____

Holding yourself accountable for your actions is a major step in your recovery. However, emotions and a fear of being judged can keep you from doing so. Ask yourself: does *not* holding yourself accountable make you happy? Usually the answer is a resounding no. Generally, denying or not taking responsibility for these behaviors only perpetuates the vicious cycle that you're trying to break free from. Let's turn now to the emotions that fuel these behaviors.

THE EMOTIONAL SOUP

The behaviors associated with BED and CO can be a way of responding to intense, often painful emotions that are difficult to cope with in any other way. Most often, we see our emotions as a problem that we have to find a solution for, and find it quick! When your emotions are in charge, you are in the emotional soup—you're blinded by your emotions and will act from them without realizing often what you are doing or saying. When you act from your emotions, you often don't think of the consequences; rather you are just concerned with relieving the discomfort caused by your emotions.

In chapter 5, we discussed DBT skills that will help you tolerate emotional distress and regulate your emotions better. Learning to be more mindfully aware of what you are feeling can reduce your risk of bingeing or overeating in response to your emotions. In the exercise below, think about situations where you've been in the emotional soup. Observe the consequences of having allowed your emotions to take over.

Identifying When You Are in the Emotional Soup

On the following list, mark the signs that tell you your emotions have taken over (write in any additional signs below). Your emotions are in the driver's seat when:

You know you shouldn't say or do something but can't stop yourself

You get so worked up you can't calm yourself down

You can't stop thinking about a situation; you obsess about it over and over

You have trouble focusing on anything else even when you are no longer in the upsetting situation

You keep telling other people about what happened to you

You just can't forget what happened

You experience physical sensations such as a racing heartbeat, sweating, flushing, or panic attacks whenever you think about the situation

People tell you that you seem moody

You can't sleep because you're so upset

Your bingeing worsens or you overeat more, even after the situation is over

_____

_____

_____

_____

When you're in the emotional soup, what you can do to help yourself feel better is:

Go for a really hard workout at the gym

Call your therapist or talk to a wise friend who will be honest with you

Journal

Go to a funny movie to distract yourself

Take a hot (or cold) shower

Do something that makes you feel good about yourself

Take a nap

_____

_____

_____

_____

Managing your emotions will give you self-confidence and a sense of security. When you're controlled by your emotions, life can be chaotic and unpredictable. Days on end can be ruined because of something that happened at home or work or school. Once you are caught in this emotional trap, you may even begin to have emotions about your emotions (e.g., you may become depressed or angry about being depressed). Being in the emotional soup is a no-win situation—but it can be overcome. In the next section we'll discuss how you can interrupt this vicious cycle.

SENSATE LAYER: BEING OPEN TO YOUR BODY'S CUES

You may have already recognized how disconnected you are from your body. In chapter 7, we'll discuss in more detail how this may have happened and what can be done about it. Right now, we'll focus on the connections between your emotions, what you feel in your body, and the behaviors associated with your BED or CO.

Physical sensations are a key part of the body's masterful design; they provide clues to all that is happening in your world. Although you may not always be aware of it, the body reliably telegraphs signals to you about what you are feeling, whether a person or situation is harmful or not, and what it needs to be healthy and feel good (food, sleep, relaxation, fun). Let's explore some of these cues with the following exercise.

Recognizing Your Body's Clues and Cues

List below the physical sensations associated with your emotions. Think of a situation in which you felt the emotion very strongly and imagine yourself standing in front of a mirror. Can you recognize what your body is feeling? Record below the emotion, physical sensation, and an example situation:

Emotion	Physical Sensation	Situation in Which You Felt This Emotion
Example: *Anger*	*My shoulders feel tight, my face flushes*	*I got turned down for a promotion*
Fear		
Guilt		
Anger		
Hurt		
Shame		
Other:		

Now, using these same emotions and situations, list the behaviors that resulted:

Emotion	Behaviors
Example: *Anger*	*I stopped at the Chinese takeout on the way home and then went home and ate too much*
Fear	
Guilt	
Anger	
Hurt	
Shame	
Other:	

The preceding exercise obviously doesn't include every human emotion, but rather, only the ones that most people don't like to feel—the ones that we try hardest to suppress. Emotions are felt in the body first. If you can realize that you're angry or hurt by recognizing the physical cue of a tingling in your stomach (or whatever your individual cue is), over time you will develop the ability to interrupt the momentum of your emotions and hence the behaviors associated with your BED or CO.

These behaviors aren't the only ones that emotions can lead to. If you ignore cues that you are angry, you may yell at your child, hang up on your girlfriend, or create some other kind of disturbance. These behaviors in the external world reflect what is going on in your internal world. Listening to your body can reduce the negative consequences of unexpressed emotions. The sensations of your body form the key to unlocking your emotions and getting yourself out of the emotional soup.

CORE BELIEFS

Core beliefs are beliefs related to a primal or core human need—the need for acceptance, love, nurturance, shelter, or protection—usually formed in times of great emotional upheaval. These beliefs tend to be a response to a problem in your life. For example, if your father died, you moved away from the town you grew up in, and your mother became depressed and withdrawn, you might have felt lost and alone, as if your life were out of control. As a result, you may have turned to food for comfort, seeking out the foods you enjoyed before all the changes in your life. In the process, you may have developed a core belief that "food is love." Or, if you were abused as a child, you may have unconsciously gained weight either to appear less attractive or to feel more powerful than you did when you were harmed. Losing weight would directly conflict with either of these core beliefs. (Core beliefs will be discussed in greater detail in chapter 8.)

Whatever your core beliefs, they may now stand in the way of your ability to recover from BED or CO. If food has become your best friend, how can you change your relationship with food without feeling lonely and deprived? You may have struggled with these feelings when you've dieted or tried to change your eating patterns in the past. In the next exercise, begin to identify how your core beliefs are connected to your behaviors, emotions, and physical sensations (you'll work further on identifying your core beliefs in chapter 8).

Identifying Barriers to Success

Think of a time when you worked hard to recover from your BED or CO, whether through therapy, nutrition counseling, dieting, or medication. Look for connections between this situation and the emotions, physical sensations, and core beliefs that kept you from achieving your goal; if you were successful but later relapsed into your old behaviors, use this experience to answer the following questions:

Describe the situation. (Example: *After I attended my sister's wedding, I decided it was time for me to stop bingeing.*)

_____

_____

_____

_____

What was your motivation to change at the time? (Example: *I couldn't believe that on what should have been a happy day, I spent most of my time sneaking food and trying not to get caught bingeing.*)

_____

_____

_____

_____

What emotions do you remember feeling then? (Example: *I was so happy for my sister, but I was ashamed because I was also jealous. I was afraid that I'd never be able to find someone who loved me like that.*)

_____

_____

_____

_____

Describe any physical sensations you felt: (Example: _My stomach was full of butterflies. There was a tightness in my chest._)

_____

_____

_____

What action did you take to stop bingeing or overeating? (Example: _I joined Weight Watchers because I had been successful with their program in the past._)

_____

_____

_____

What you learned from this exercise is that one of your greatest fears is: (Example: _That no one will care about me and I'll be alone._)

_____

_____

_____

The core belief you've formed because of this fear is: (Example: _I must look a certain way for someone to love me._)

_____

_____

_____

_____

As you're starting to see, the behaviors associated with your BED or CO are part of a greater chain. Becoming more aware of the connections between the different links of this chain will make you better able to break it at any point along the way. It may take some time to become skilled at breaking the pattern in its early stages. This is a two-step process that requires first being mindfully aware of your emotions, physical sensations, and beliefs—this can take practice. The second step is recognizing that you have the ability to choose whether to continue the pattern and its behaviors. When you choose, you also hold yourself accountable for your choice.

THE DEEPER URGES OF THE SOUL

Beneath all of the superficial behaviors, emotional soup, physical sensations, and core beliefs is a code much like the genetic code of your DNA. However, this code is the code of your soul or spirit. While your genetic code may make you more prone to being overweight, your soul code is what makes you want to become a parent. It's what pulls you toward a career in teaching or medicine or law. It's what directs you to climb mountains or aid the homeless. It's what helps you soar to greater heights, motivating you when you feel like quitting. It's what inspires you to be a good person or kind to a stranger. It is the healthy part of you—the part that wants to see you recover and move on with your life.

Right now, much of your soul code may be buried under the weight of your BED/CO. Even though you may have achieved some of the goals you've set yourself, as long as so much of your energy is devoted to satisfying the demands of your eating disorder, it will be difficult for you to experience true happiness or joy. When you relate directly to life itself through your soul code, you'll find that what you have previously considered your best or happiest times do not compare to the happiness and joy your life now holds for you. In the past, food may have served as your comfort. Now, in recovery, your soul self will anchor you through the storms of life.

The Deeper Urges of Your Soul

List the five things you value most in your life: (Example: My *family, my pets, my faith, my children, and giving back to others.*)

1. _____

2. _____

3. _____

4. _____

5. _____

List five things you had hoped to do in your life when you were younger, things you dreamed about: (Example: *I dreamed of working as a missionary in a third world country.*)

1. _____

2. _____

3. _____

4. _____

5. _____

Describe the emotions and thoughts that arise when you think about your dreams and the things that are most important to you in your life: (Example: *I had forgotten some of the goals I once had. I feel sad that my life is so focused on my eating problems rather than on what's most important to me. This makes me feel even more motivated to make changes.*)

_____

_____

_____

_____

_____

The deeper urges of the soul self are difficult to "hear" when buried under years of BED/CO behaviors, emotions, sensations, and beliefs. But beneath everything, your soul self awaits you. As you read on, layer by layer your soul code will be revealed. As you work through the rest of the book, pay attention for signs of the deeper urges of the soul. Continue to write in your journal about new insights and changes in your thought processes and emotional expression, but now also write about this important emergence of the soul's deeper urges.

ED SELF VS. SOUL SELF

It's important to see the difference between your ED (eating disorder) self or unhealthy self and your soul self or non-ED self. (Think of these as two separate parts of yourself: "ED me" and "non-ED me.") Your unhealthy ED self includes characteristics from all the levels we've just discussed. Its behaviors include binge eating or compulsive overeating as well as behaviors such as drug abuse, gambling, lying, and so on. It is the personification of your emotional soup and the physical sensations that lurk beneath it. It is where your core beliefs hold sway over you, keeping you from your true dreams and goals. Think of your ED self as a character in a play—a character whose personality is based on certain life experiences, who feels certain types of emotions more than others and has core beliefs formed by the past.

Beneath the ED self is the soul self yearning for expression. The soul self is the essence of who you are, the part of you that never changes—your intellect, your passions, your innate beauty and humanity. The soul self speaks the language of love and acceptance and is as close to you as your heart. The ED self, on the other hand, often has a harsh, judgmental tongue that tells you to doubt yourself and increases your suffering.

The purpose of separating your ED self from your soul self or non-ED self is to give you some distance from the negative judgments and emotions that can keep you stuck in the emotional soup. Dump everything that has led to your BED/CO into your ED self. In the end, this false self must cede to your soul self. We all have different parts of ourselves; in the case of individuals with BED/CO, the false ED self may have taken over and may now be more in evidence than the true self.

ED Self vs. Soul Self

On one side of the following chart, list qualities, emotions, appearance, and fears to describe your false, ED self—list anything that helps you capture what it is like. On the other side, list qualities of your true, soul self. (I've provided an example to help you get started.)

Characteristics of Your ED Self (ED Me)	Characteristics of Your Soul Self (non-ED Me)
I am overweight and disgusting	I have good friends who care about me
I like to be in control	I am a good parent
Emotions: guilt, shame, fear, anger	I am curious, adventurous, and kind
I will do anything to get people to like me	I am very compassionate
My thighs are too big	
I am not a good father	
I'm a failure—I feel alone and lonely and I don't have any close friends	
I know people judge me because of how I look so I've decided to flaunt it and wear revealing clothes	

In writing this example, I have deliberately not filled up the space for characteristics of the soul self, because for many of you it may take some time to remember who you really are. To do this, try going through old photo albums. One of my patients saw from old pictures of herself how spunky she was, always wearing bright colors and eye-catching bracelets. As she began to remember her spirit, she realized how her compulsive overeating and the life experiences that led to her eating disorder had buried it.

Characteristics of Your ED Self (ED Me)	Characteristics of Your Soul Self (non-ED Me)

You can expand this exercise by putting old photos and magazine clippings—both words and pictures work—that remind you of your soul self either in your journal or somewhere easy to see on a daily basis.

I cannot emphasize enough how important it is for you to begin to recognize the patterns and connections that drive your BED or CO. Only by becoming aware of how your eating disorder is currently holding you hostage can you hope to break free. Becoming more aware is akin to shining a flashlight into a dark cave: The more aware you are, the brighter the light becomes—and the less scary the cave seems. Eventually, you can explore your entire life without judgment, recognizing that while certain events may have taken you off course, you can still find your way.

Know that although the deepest, most important urges of your healthy self may presently be hidden beneath layers that support your BED/CO, your soul level is still very strong—if not, you would not be reading this book. Keep shining the light on what matters most to you and you will find the inspiration and knowledge that will give you the strength to complete your journey to recovery.

SUMMARY

By now you should have a clearer picture of who you are when you engage in your BED/CO—its set of associated behaviors, physical sensations, and core beliefs that formed in response to the pain of being human and your own particular life experiences.

As you continue on your journey to recovery, you'll begin to see shifts in these levels. Over time, your soul self will return to the top to direct your emotions and physical sensations and help you form healthy new core beliefs. You'll know this is happening when you no longer engage in bingeing, overeating, and the other behaviors associated with your BED/CO. These behaviors will be replaced by actions that support your recovery and move you toward greater fulfillment in your life. You'll also no longer get stuck as often in the emotional soup; instead, you'll be better able to recognize your emotions and their associated physical sensations and, using the skills you're learning in this book, interrupt any unhealthy behaviors. Your core beliefs will then support your passion in life and no longer be a barrier to your recovery.

CHAPTER 7

Mirror, Mirror

written with Isabelle Tierney, MA, LMFT, BHSP

If you struggle with BED or CO, you probably also struggle with a negative body image. You may wish your body were different—better, thinner—and may feel very frustrated by its imperfections. You may imagine that a perfect body would bring you happiness, and you may work endlessly, though fruitlessly, to make that dream a reality.

BODY IMAGE

What is *body image*? Your body image is your mental picture of what your body looks like. It is the collection of thoughts and feelings you have about how your body looks, not a description of how your body really is. It is a conclusion about your body that came about by comparing it to other bodies. Constant comparison—particularly with images from the media—can make you feel imperfect and can lead to negative body image and body-destructive actions like bingeing or overeating.

If you are dissatisfied with your body, you are not alone. Body dissatisfaction is felt by millions of people in the United States—dissatisfaction directed toward both our own bodies and the less than perfect bodies of others. In one survey, 59 percent of young girls expressed dissatisfaction with their body shape and 66 percent expressed the desire to lose weight (Field et al. 1999); disturbingly, older women are also increasingly being diagnosed with eating disorders.

Loving Your Body

The first step toward greater satisfaction with your body is to stop seeing your body as a separate entity to be controlled and manipulated. Your relationship with your body is your very first relationship. You come into the world with your body and you go out with your body. Your body is the longest-lasting friend you have, and it performs miracles for you on a daily basis. It has helped you survive illness, injury, and other difficult times. It may have even given birth to a child. Your body may also have survived abuse, trauma, or addiction. Your body supports you right now, and continues to support you as you struggle with BED or CO—your heart beats, your lungs inhale and exhale, and your muscles stretch and contract and take you places. When you learn to love, protect, and care for your body, you learn basic skills that will improve not only your relationship with yourself—which is very important—but your relationship with other people as well.

THE FIVE RELATIONAL SKILLS

The remainder of this chapter explores how to develop a healthy relationship with your body by moving from an external focus (your image of your body) to an internal focus (being in a relationship with your body). You will learn five relationship skills: active attention, listening, communicating, give and take, and active loving. These skills will help you to truly know and love your body. Work with the skills thoroughly and patiently—each skill builds upon earlier ones and is a lifelong practice on its own. This work will bring you more gifts than you ever expected. Enjoy them!

Skill 1: Establishing Contact with Your Body Through Active Attention

When you struggle with body image issues, you rarely see your body for what it is. You see the surface but miss the depth and wonder inside. Active attention acts as an antidote to such distorted vision. With active attention, you expand your focus beyond surface appearance to the whole body, inside and out. This helps you shift your perception of your body. No longer is your body an object to be bullied by perfectionism, now it is a life-filled entity with unlimited potential.

Active attention requires curiosity and a willingness to take the time to truly get to know your partner—your body. Active attention is different from looking in the mirror and repetitively thinking, "My thighs have cellulite," or, "My stomach is fat." With active attention, you suspend judgment and begin to search for deeper truths. You take the time to investigate what's happening below the usual judgments, to connect with who your body really is. How are your intestines doing after your last binge? What are your bones and muscles telling you? What about your heart? Can you let your heart be filled with gratitude?

Learning to shift your perception of your body is not something that happens overnight. Repeat the following exercises over time to increase your awareness of how you view your body and your ability to see it with the awe and respect it deserves.

Assess Your Current Relationship With Your Body

Describe what you like most about your body (example: *I like my brown eyes*):

_____

_____

_____

_____

Describe what you like least about your body (example: *My knees are knobby*):

_____

_____

_____

_____

What do these likes and dislikes tell you about your current relationship with your body? (Example: *My list of negatives was much longer than my list of positives. This tells me I have more negative feelings about my body than I would like. Or, When I see these dislikes in writing, I'm a little ashamed that I'm so hard on myself.*)

_____

_____

_____

_____

_____

_____

For most people with BED/CO, it's easier to focus on the external appearance of the body—the way you look—rather than on internal information. This outside-in focus can cause a lot of pain, as how you look is almost never good enough. Over time, by shifting from an external focus to an internal focus, you can reduce the judgments and negative self-talk you now experience in regard to your body image.

Shifting the Relationship with Active Attention

To shift your relationship with your body, you need to see it in a different way. Focus not on a one-dimensional view of its exterior, but on its interior, its magnificence. Take charge of your perceptions—don't allow the past to dictate how you feel about your body and don't allow your dissatisfaction with your body to influence how you feel about yourself as a person. As a child—or even now as an adult—you may have felt that you weren't seen or understood for who you were but rather were judged by your appearance. If you pay close attention, you'll realize that you're actually perpetuating this pattern when you place undue attention on your physical appearance.

Shifting Your Perspective Through Active Attention

This exercise helps you begin to shift your perception of your body. Although this exercise focuses on the abdomen (an area many people are dissatisfied with), you can do it with any body part that you feel dissatisfied with.

Lie on a flat surface—perhaps your bed—and place your hand on the skin of your abdomen. Notice your immediate first thought. Usually it's a judgment. Stop yourself when you hear your mind cranking out judgments. Next, shift your attention to the hand on your belly. Notice how it feels for the skin of your hand to rest on the skin of your belly. Take a moment to thank your body's millions of skin cells that serve as a protective barrier against the harsh environment. Next, notice the rise and fall of your belly with your breath. Take a deep breath, then direct that breath with its life-giving oxygen to your belly. Give thanks to your breath for the oxygen it carries to every cell in your body. Next, imagine the muscles that lie beneath the skin and allow you to move your body. Thank them for doing this. Practice this exercise as many times as you can during the day. Write down any changes in your perception of your abdomen after doing the exercise:

_____

_____

_____

Use your journal to continue to record insights about your abdomen and other body parts.

Skill 2: Listening to Your Body

Listening seems like such a simple skill, yet few of us do it well. Listening to another is hard enough. Listening to your body is even harder, as your body's voice is neither loud nor always very clear.

When you don't listen to your body, you become stuck in a one-sided relationship and, as a result, often end up taking actions that can be very painful. If you eat before discovering if your body is actually hungry, you end up hurting your body and feeling highly uncomfortable. If you don't listen to your body's need for rest, you wind up exhausted and depleted, slowing your life down to a crawl. Ignoring your body's signals of fullness can lead to weight gain; ignoring its signals for exercise can lead to lethargy and disease. The following three steps will help you become a better listener, both to your body and others:

1. Get yourself *physically* ready to listen. It's easy to get distracted by another task while trying to listen. Unfortunately, it's just not possible to both listen deeply and do something else. Find a quiet place. Sit down, let your body get still. Open all of your senses. The body communicates through sight, sound, touch, taste, and smell.

2. Get yourself *psychologically* ready to listen. Do you really want to hear what your body has to say? When you struggle with eating issues, you're often completely disconnected from your body's needs. Your body may tell you it's not hungry while your eating disorder is urging you to devour a pint of ice cream. Taking the time to actually listen can prove disconcerting, as your body's messages may be very different from your eating disorder's.

3. Watch for common listening obstacles such as:

   * Building your argument while your body (or another person) is speaking. For example, you may feel tired and sleepy because your body is telling you it needs to rest. But in your mind you may be arguing against rest by thinking about the deadline you have at work.

   * Being stuck in judgments that prevent you from really hearing the messages of the body.

   * Being impatient. This can be especially hard, as the body often communicates both more slowly and less clearly than the mind. How often have you thought you were still hungry only to find out a few minutes later that your body had had enough?

   * Projecting information onto the body that has nothing to do with what your body has actually communicated. For example, you might tell yourself your body is hungry—because you want to eat—although your body may have communicated the exact opposite.

When learning to listen to your body, it is vital to be curious and patient. You are listening to a lifelong partner who often communicates differently than you. Can you take the time to learn your body's language, even if it's not always easy? You've probably been asked to do this at least once in your life already, whether with an infant or pet, or in a foreign country you visited on vacation. If your body is communicating its need for food through your senses, you might, for example, find yourself imagining a picture of a caesar salad, hearing the words "caesar salad," or even feeling the texture of salad as you think about chewing it.

Finally, if you aren't sure what your body is communicating, keep listening by continuing to ask your body what it needs, focusing your attention on your physical sensations, and staying as quiet as you can. Watch for interfering thoughts; if you notice any, let them go. With time, patience, and openness, you will become an expert listener!

Assess the Current Relationship Through Deep Listening

Describe a time when you listened to your body and changed what you (your mind) were going to do in order to do what your body wanted instead: (Example: *Last night my friends called me up to go out to a restaurant that has a buffet. I was very tired from work and I usually end up bingeing when I'm tired, so I decided to go home, eat, and go to bed early.*)

_____

_____

_____

_____

_____

_____

How did it feel to honor your body in this way?

_____

_____

The following exercise will help you practice listening during mealtimes by checking your body's hunger and fullness levels before you eat, while you eat, and after you eat. Although this exercise focuses on food, you can also use it to practice listening in other areas, such as to assess your body's need for rest or exercise.

Shift Your Relationship with Your Body Through Deep Listening

Do this either at your next meal or at a meal where you feel comfortable and have control over your food options, such as when you are cooking at home.

Close your eyes. Take several deep breaths. Bring your awareness to the very top of your head, then slowly begin to scan through your body, moving from your head to your neck, shoulders, arms and hands. Scan further down, into your chest, abdomen, back, and hips. Finally bring your awareness to your legs and feet.

When you feel fully present (and you'll know you are because the chatter in your mind will have slowed down) you're ready to listen to your body. Assess your body's hunger level from 1–10, with 1 being extreme hunger and 10 being extreme fullness. Circle the number that applies:

1   2   3   4   5   6   7   8   9   10

Ask your body what it needs to eat. Be open to your body's language: it could show you images, vocalize words, or communicate through body sensations. If you don't get clear information, offer it different types of food by thinking of words or images of particular foods, then listen to how your body responds. Write down the messages you get from your body below:

_____

_____

_____

_____

Check in with your body throughout the meal. It's often hardest to listen to your intuition at mealtimes, as your body is slower than your mind to let you know when it's had enough. Use the 1–10 scale to assess your fullness level:

1   2   3   4   5   6   7   8   9   10

Describe how your body felt after this meal:

_____

_____

_____

_____

Skill 3: Communication with Your Body

Communication is a vital aspect of any relationship, often determining the quality of a relationship. Communicate with love and respect and you create a healthy and thriving relationship. Communicate with shame and bitterness and the relationship flounders. Communicating with your body is no different.

If you are a binge eater, you may have experienced critical communication from others in childhood, including harsh judgments, shaming words, and put-downs. You may have internalized this negative style of communication, and use it now yourself to communicate with your body. How others, such as peers, the media, and authority figures such as teachers, coaches, or even bosses, communicate—both with others and with their bodies—can also strongly impact you. It is difficult to speak lovingly to your body when most of the people around you talk hatefully about their own bodies or the bodies of other people. After all, will you still be accepted if you tell them you love your body?

The way you talk to your body has profound ramifications for both your physical and psychological health. Thoughts and emotions influence the very cells in your body. Sad or negative thoughts cause your brain to produce neurotransmitters that weaken your immune system; thoughts of hostility induce rapid heartbeat and heightened blood pressure; anxious thoughts can raise your blood pressure (Rosenkranz et al. 2003). On the other hand, thoughts and feelings of happiness, love, and compassion actually produce physiological changes that lead to better health. This is because these feelings generate neurotransmitters that then stimulate the immune system and increase resistance to disease (Matsunaga et al. 2008).

The following exercises will help you understand how you're currently communicating with your body and offer strategies for more loving communication. Rather than criticizing and judging your body, use words of gratitude and appreciation. Use the same mushy, unselfconscious words when referring to your body that you'd use to express your love to a child, a beloved pet, or to other loved ones.

We are often unaware of how we speak to our bodies because the words are not spoken out loud and usually pass just below our consciousness. As you start bringing these words into your consciousness, you'll find they create a lot of emotional pain. Be kind to yourself—immediately switch to loving words, even if you don't fully believe them yet.

Assess the Current Relationship Through Communication

List the three most common statements you make about your body. These may be statements that come up before meals, when you're around someone you feel insecure with, when you're feeling sad or tired, or when you weigh yourself or look in the mirror:

_____

_____

_____

_____

Imagine that you are in a foreign land and have no preconceived notions about how the people there feel about their bodies. If you heard people in this foreign country say the three statements listed above over and over, how would you interpret it? What would you assume they felt about their bodies?

_____

_____

_____

_____

Next, let's focus on shifting your relationship with your body by changing how you communicate with your body.

Shift the Relationship Through Communication

For the next three days, practice changing your style of communication with your body.

When you notice you're speaking negatively to your body, *stop*. Walk away, distract yourself, do something that feels good. Even if you can't automatically shift to loving communication yet, just stopping negative communication can lead to huge changes.

Next, use more loving communication, even if it feels forced. If you were thinking how fat your stomach was, shift your perception to see your body differently. Put your hand on your stomach and imagine your skin cells, your intestines, or your spine. Spend a minute or two really connecting with these body parts, observing how hard they work for you, how alive they are. As your heart opens, tell your body how grateful you are. This can help rewire your brain physiology, with a huge impact your mind and body.

After you've practiced loving communication toward your body for one full day, describe how this feels in the space below. You may feel embarrassed or think the exercise is stupid. Any emotion or thought is all right as long as you continue to practice loving communication. Use your journal to track how your feelings about your body—or doing this exercise—change over time.

_____

_____

_____

_____

_____

Skill 4: Give and Take

What happens when you've listened to your body and realized that it needs something, but this something is very different from what your mind says you need? For example, if you've just worked out, your body may crave protein while your mind is dying for warm chocolate chip cookies as a reward for your hard efforts. Or your body may tell you it's full while your mind wants you to keep eating. Before, when you didn't listen to your body, it was much easier to do what exactly what your mind wanted. Now that you're listening and learning to communicate with your body, you have to decide how to take what your body needs into account.

This is no different from any other relationship. It is very normal to experience conflicting needs in a relationship. Some of these are simple—for example, you may want to see a movie while your partner wants to take a nap. Others are more complex—your partner may want to move to Hawaii while you're certain you'd die away from New York. How do you handle conflicting needs? Do you usually yield to the needs of others, or do you meet your needs first? Are you a giver or a taker? The way you were raised can influence how you handle conflicting needs. You may have been raised to take others' needs into account first. Alternatively, you may have learned as a child to take care of yourself first.

Either way, negotiating between your mind and your body doesn't always have to be a win/lose proposition, it can be win/win. What does the win/win choice look like? Here are a couple of examples:

* You feed your body protein and *then* have chocolate chip cookies. Thus, you give your body what it needs but still nurture your emotional self. Deprivation does not even enter your mind as you know you'll get what you want.

* You have your cookies first, but kindly promise your body you'll feed it protein later. This creates balance in the system and gives you a nourished body that can support you in your life.

In either case, *both* entities in the relationship are taken into account—something that doesn't usually happen when in the middle of a typical binge or day of overeating.

Think of the give and take skill as negotiating give and take between your child self and your adult self or your mind and your body. Both are true. What matters most is recognizing the need to both give and take—don't approach your relationship with your body as an all-or-nothing situation.

Assess the Current Relationship Through Give and Take

What happens when your body and your mind want different things? For example, let's say your body tells you it wants greens while your mind really wants ice cream. What's your immediate reaction? If you are in a safe situation, say it out loud. (Example: *I don't care what you want. I want what I want when I want it, regardless of the consequences.*) Bringing this voice into consciousness and being truthful gives you an honest mirror of who you are in the relationship. This allows you to decide whether your current role in the relationship is good enough for you or whether you want to make changes.

Think of a time when your body and mind wanted very different things and answer the following questions:

What did your mind want?

_____

_____

_____

If you did what your mind wanted, what happened? How did your body feel? Your mind?

_____

_____

If you did what your body wanted, what happened? How did your body feel? Your mind?

_____

_____

_____

What can you honestly see yourself doing differently when handling the conflicting needs of your mind and body in the future?

_____

_____

_____

Sometimes you may feel torn between satisfying emotional or mental needs and taking care of your body. If so, remind yourself that emotional needs often represent other needs that were never satisfied in childhood. Satisfying them now in the same way you did as a child—e.g., eating to fill the emotional void of your mother's death or to comfort you after being bullied at school—will not ultimately be satisfying. What "worked" in childhood no longer works for you as an adult—and can create significant health problems. Let's practice the give and take skill.

Shift the Relationship Through Give and Take

Practice give and take at your next meal. Using loving communication, make it clear to your body and mind that both your emotional and your physical needs will be met, though not necessarily at the same time. (Example: _I will eat cake now but I promise to give you protein and vegetables later tonight._) Describe what you decided to do and how it felt to practice give and take:

_____

_____

_____

_____

Skill 5: Active Loving

How often do you act lovingly toward your body? If you struggle with binge eating or compulsive overeating, the punishing cycle of bingeing and dieting is probably closer to a relationship from hell than to a loving partnership. You may be focused on controlling your body rather than loving it. This can lead to pain and emptiness, as it often conflicts with the urges of your soul self, the essence of who you are.

With active loving you treat your body as if you are falling in love with it. You romance your body by showing it—through specific actions—that you regard it with the awe and reverence that it deserves. You make it feel appreciated, supported, valued, and enjoyed.

You may initially resist acting lovingly toward your body. Do it anyway. As said in twelve-step groups, "act as if" and "fake it until you make it." When you practice acts of kindness, you connect to your heart and your soul, engaging them to work for you. The more often you practice active loving, the easier it becomes—until you wake up one day and realize that loving-kindness has become an integral part of your life.

Gratitude—Three Practices

1. Throughout the day, as often as you can, express instant gratitude to your body. For example, you might thank your kidneys when you go to the bathroom or your leg muscles when you walk somewhere. Record these thoughts of gratitude in your journal every day.

2. Every month—every week if you can—create a celebration day for your body. Act as though it's your body's birthday. How do you treat people on their birthday? You think about them, do kind things for them, buy them presents, and celebrate their uniqueness. Birthday parties may usually make you think of bingeing on cake and ice cream or indulging in all the sweets you want to eat. However, because it is unlikely that your body will thrive for long periods of time on cake or ice cream, find other fun and enjoyable ways to celebrate your body besides with food. The following suggestions will get you started:

   Give your body a massage

   Eat lots of fruits and vegetables

   Put your body first in every food decision you make

   _____

   _____

   _____

   _____

3. Buy—or borrow from your library—a book that describes how your anatomy works. Then, at least once a week learn something new about your body. You live with your body every day—getting to really know it is one of the most loving gifts you can do. Start by listing six things you've learned about your body: (Example: *I learned that every second ten million cells die and are replaced in my body.*)

_____

_____

_____

_____

_____

_____

REPAIR AND HEALING

If you have BED or CO, you may have used guilt and shame to try to stop behaviors you are not proud of. You may have deprived yourself of things, or punished yourself for not sticking to a diet or exercise plan. If you overeat, you may have starved yourself for a week or exercised excessively to make up for the harm—real or imagined—you've done yourself. These kinds of behaviors perpetuate the self-destructive cycle of body dissatisfaction, low self-esteem, shame, and guilt. Guilt is driven by your mind, by a harsh inner critic with narrow definitions of what's right and wrong. This critic wants to punish you with rigid consequences that have nothing to do with what's actually needed in the moment. Guilt promotes stress in the body rather than healing.

How do you break this cycle? How do you take responsibility for your actions if you don't use guilt as a motivator? By practicing remorse instead of guilt. Remorse arises from the heart. It requires you to fully take another into account, to empathize with him, to fully feel the effect of your actions upon his well-being. You soften rather than harden, and as a result can be flexible in your actions. With remorse, there are no rigid rules. Rather, remorse only requires that you stay present with your body's needs, that you be willing to compassionately ask your body what it needs. Because remorse arises from your heart, choices that support your health and well-being automatically spring forth.

But how does remorse differ from guilt in real life? Let's say you binged last night. As a result, today when you wake up, you are filled with guilt and shame. Your critic berates you, criticizing your body even more than usual, calling it fat, ugly, and embarrassing. You resolve to be "good" today, committing to eating only 500 calories and going on a three-hour bike ride. In the moment of committing, you feel great. You have a tough plan of action and the inner critic is momentarily appeased. Unfortunately, your plan isn't connected to your body's needs, so you are bingeing again by the middle of the day.

With remorse, you first take responsibility for your actions and apologize for them—authentically, just as if you had lost your temper with a loved one. This isn't the "I'm sorry" you say to get someone off your back, but the "I'm sorry" that truly takes into account the hurt you caused—in this case to your body, your stomach, and your intestines. Then, you check in with your body, lovingly ask it how it feels. Don't assume anything. Be present to whatever your body is telling you. This will feel much better than guilt, and will serve both you and your body at the highest level.

Guilt-inspired action has nothing to do with what your body truly needs. Remorseful action does. With remorse, you can acknowledge that your child self may have needed to turn to food to feel loved or cared for, while recognizing that as an adult there are healthier skills you can use to cope with your emotional needs. Remorse helps you to repair and heal your relationship with your body.

Use the following exercise to practice repair and healing. Remember: your goal is to develop healthy skills that will help you end the cycle of guilt, shame, and punishment. You probably either learned these behaviors as a child or developed them out of a mistaken sense that guilt, shame, and punishment would motivate you to change your bingeing or overeating. Now that you are aware that this cycle is self-destructive, you can shift your relationship to your body and begin to repair and heal the damage this cycle has done to you.

Repair and Healing

Observe how you treat your body after you binge or overeat. Observe how—whether—you listen to it, how you communicate with it, how you punish or forgive it. Observe, too, how often you repeat the same pattern. List any statements you made or actions you took after you last binged or overate: (Example: *I try not to eat for a whole day if I've binged.*)

_____

_____

_____

_____

_____

What emotions do you experience when you think about these statements and actions?

_____

_____

Take a moment to think about the skills you've learned in this chapter that you could practice after you binge or overeat. (The skills you learned in this chapter are: active attention, deep listening, communication, give and take, and active loving.) List skills you could have used in this situation:

_____

_____

_____

_____

_____

_____

SUMMARY

Developing a healthy relationship with your body is a lifelong process. Just as you never stop practicing relationship skills with family and friends, it is vital to keep practicing relationship skills with your body. The five relationship skills described in this chapter will help you shift from an unhealthy relationship with your body to a more loving partnership. As you practice these skills, you'll find other relationships will heal as well. These skills apply to any relationship—the more you listen to your body, the better you'll be able to listen to others; the more you communicate lovingly with your body, the more you'll communicate lovingly with others; and so on. Keep practicing, and enjoy learning to be in a loving relationship with your oldest best friend—your body.

CHAPTER 8

Challenging Your Core Beliefs

At times, you may have sincerely wanted to change your behaviors but ended up frustrated because you were unable to stop bingeing or overeating despite your best efforts. You may have even said to yourself, "Something seems to be in my way." If so, you were probably right: core beliefs that you are not consciously aware of may be blocking your progress toward your desired goal.

But these unhealthy core beliefs don't have to control you. When you understand what they are and how they developed, you can change them—and replace them with healthy guiding principles that will help the new you flourish.

WHAT ARE CORE BELIEFS?

A *core belief* is a doctrine or rule about life that usually develops in response to a situation in which you feel your survival is threatened or for which you do not have adequate coping skills. Core beliefs are often formed in childhood or during intense emotional or traumatic experiences.

For example, if your parents divorce when you're nine and your relationship with one of them is severed, you may feel overwhelming emotions that you can't handle at that age. So you'll cope the best you can, developing a rule to keep your feelings under control. This rule may be "never let anyone see me upset" or "when I eat [a comfort food], I don't feel so upset." At the time, this rule "saves" you, at least emotionally. However, as you can imagine, this same rule will cause multiple problems when you grow up.

As you grow older, you may no longer be aware of these core beliefs. As a result, you may be acting from beliefs that no longer serve you—or in fact are counter to your current wishes and needs. Thus core beliefs, although they may have served a very important purpose when initially formed, may sabotage your ability to change later in life.

Before eliminating outdated core beliefs, it is important to understand how the belief or beliefs served you in the past, because part of you is still using these beliefs for that same purpose. Imagine you were able to surgically remove your outdated core beliefs—how would the needs they address be met? Let's look at an example of how core beliefs are formed and how they can affect a person throughout his life.

Tony's Story

At thirty-six, Tony has struggled with compulsive overeating since his early teens. Tony was not overweight as a child—just the opposite: he had asthma and was skinny and sickly until his teen years. As a result, his mother worried about his health and pampered him. She prepared special food for him and didn't allow him to get overheated or exert himself too much. When Tony and his older brother Mike got into mischief, Mike was always punished while Tony was just told to go to his room. This increased normal sibling rivalry to the point where Tony's brother often "punished" Tony in private, beating him up when their mother wasn't around.

Over time, Tony grew taller and heavier than Mike. Then, during one of their arguments, Tony actually tore Mike's bedroom door off its hinges in a fit of rage, and Mike was, for the first time, frightened of Tony. From that moment on, Mike could no longer beat him up. For the first time in his life, Tony felt more powerful than his older brother.

Later, in treatment as an adult for his compulsive overeating—which had resulted in his becoming obese and developing diabetes and high blood pressure—Tony recalled this experience. The core beliefs Tony had formed during childhood experiences like this one were making it difficult for him to be happy and healthy as an adult. Tony was able to identify two problematic core beliefs.

CORE BELIEF 1: I NEED TO BE IN MY COMFORT ZONE TO FEEL SAFE

Tony's comfort zone consisted of a narrow range of behaviors and emotions; when he wasn't in it, he felt afraid and anxious without understanding why. During his childhood, his mother had always emphasized that he needed to avoid overexerting himself or getting upset to prevent an asthma attack. In Tony's mind, staying comfortable was associated with safety. His reaction to being outside his comfort zone was to immediately retreat. For example, because he felt very uncomfortable with expressing anger, whenever he became angry, he would suppress his anger by overeating. In his marriage, any changes or conflict that pushed him out of his comfort zone led to feelings of resentment. He felt that his wife didn't understand and accept him, and that he wasn't good enough for her because he couldn't meet her expectations.

CORE BELIEF 2: BIGGER IS BETTER

In Tony's mind, his ability to intimidate his brother was closely linked to his new size. At sixteen, he was finally bigger than Mike, no longer vulnerable to Mike's fists. As an adult, when Tony dieted and successfully lost weight, his smaller size made him feel physically vulnerable again, and he would regain his weight. In his marriage, although unable to match his wife's income, Tony unconsciously tried to equalize the power differential by literally being bigger than his wife. This core belief—bigger is better—was thus sabotaging his ability to achieve what he really wanted: to have a healthy body, be a strong partner in his marriage, and feel good about himself.

For Tony, becoming aware of his core beliefs allowed him to identify the many areas of his life they were unconsciously influencing. This helped him understand why he found himself unable to accomplish goals he felt sincerely committed to.

Let's explore now how and why core beliefs develop. This will help you identify the important purposes various core beliefs have served in your life.

How Core Beliefs Develop

Although Tony's story may have given you a sense of how core beliefs form, you may still have more questions than answers. Some important things to remember about core beliefs:

* When they first form, core beliefs serve a specific purpose or fill a need

* Core beliefs are formed during difficult or emotional times in our lives

* Core beliefs often become unconscious

* All of us have core beliefs that we have forgotten about but which are on autopilot—we continue to act from these beliefs whether we know it or not

For example, if you grew up in a family with a father who was a violent alcoholic, you may have tried to protect yourself from uncertainty and abuse by becoming a tough kid—and later a tough adult. A core belief you may have developed is that letting people get close to you only leads to pain. Even though the purpose this coping behavior once served—to protect yourself—may no longer be relevant, the behaviors that support the core belief may continue.

What Purpose Do Your Core Beliefs Serve?

If you were the tough kid described above, your core belief would keep others from getting close to you, preventing the kind of constant disappointment you felt with your alcoholic parent. However, you might also forget the primary desire that inspired this pain: your desire to be close to your father. (Although you may feel intense anger toward him, beneath that anger is probably sadness and loss.) Once the core belief is in place it will work very hard on your behalf to protect you from pain. Even if your father re-enters your life, you may find yourself so shut down that you are not able to reconnect with the primal need to be close to him. Thus, keeping people away—being the tough kid and later the tough adult—also keeps you from having what you really want: close relationships with your father and others.

Core beliefs can also form as a result of neglect. If you had an alcoholic parent like our tough kid, you may have been neglected as a child, forming the core belief that you have to take care of yourself because no one else will. As you grew up, you may have become very competent—perhaps so competent that others become intimidated or feel they cannot make a meaningful contribution to your life—or very stressed and overwhelmed, feeling as if you always have to do everything on your own. Such feelings of stress can then lead to unhealthy coping behaviors.

Now that you have a better understanding of what core beliefs are, and how and why they form, let's discuss first, how to identify core beliefs, and second, how these beliefs may impact your BED/CO.

IDENTIFYING YOUR CORE BELIEFS

Core beliefs tend to be related to fundamental human needs—for love, acceptance, respect, support, self-expression, empowerment, and to be heard. These needs and the circumstances that surround them are all clues to your core beliefs. Follow these clues to identify your core beliefs. You may also already have some ideas about what your core beliefs are. You'll know when you actually hit on a core belief, as you'll have the sense that you've discovered something quite profound that explains many of the issues you've been struggling with.

Clue 1: Major Life Events You've Experienced

Major life events are often pivotal, as they may change many aspects of our lives and our perceptions. Thinking back on these events, you may realize that you became different somehow after the event occurred. In this difference lies the nugget of truth that will guide you to any core beliefs that may have formed.

Major Life Events

The following are some major, but common life events you may have experienced. Circle those that apply to you, adding any others in the extra lines provided below:

* Your parents divorced when you were age _____.

* One or both of your parents was an alcoholic or drug addict.

* One or both of your parents suffered from a chronic illness when you were a child.

    * Chronic depression or other mental illness (schizophrenia, anxiety, obsessive-compulsive disorder)

    * Cancer

    * Other major medical problem _____

* A loved one died. This person was: _____.

* You were molested or abused (physically, sexually, or emotionally) as a child.

* You were neglected as a child (your primary caretaker left you alone for long periods when very young or did not fulfill basic needs for food, shelter, emotional connection).

* You were abandoned or felt abandoned by one of your parents.

* You were bullied or in some way shamed and threatened by another person who was older, bigger, or in a position of authority. Describe: _____

_____

_____ .

* Other events:

_____

_____

_____

_____

Clue 2: Your Interpretation of What Happened to You and How You Coped

Choose the two events from the previous exercise that seem most significant to you. As you look over the events, notice any emotions or physical sensations you feel, even if fleeting. Examine closely any events that still hold a strong emotional or sensory charge, and any events that set your mind racing with memories. These are the ones you want to focus on for the purposes of this exercise. You'll work with these two events for the remaining exercises in this chapter.

Caution: If you have untreated trauma in your past, do not work with your traumatic experience as it may trigger memories or flashbacks. Choose a less emotional experience to start with. For any choice, if emotions surface that you cannot control, stop the exercise and seek professional help immediately.

How You Coped with Your Experiences

Describe the two events/experiences without trying to analyze what happened. Try to remember what this experience was like for you at the time you went through it.

Example:

Target experience: *My mother had chronic depression when I was growing up.*

How you coped: *I tried to not make a lot of noise when I got home from school if my mom was having one of her sick days. I would make lunches for my sister and myself and sometimes we would eat peanut butter sandwiches every night for dinner if Mom was not well. I tried not to bring her any of my problems because I didn't want to upset her. I brought special treats to her room—cookies and milk, sandwiches, or pictures I drew for her—to try to cheer her up. I always tried to put on a happy face around her.*

Target experience A:

_____

_____

How you coped:

_____

_____

_____

_____

_____

_____

Target experience B:

_____

_____

How you coped:

_____

_____

_____

_____

_____

_____

Later, you may also want to explore other life experiences to help you uncover additional core beliefs. Use your journal to describe other situations and how you coped.

Uncovering the Core Belief

Remember: your core beliefs usually represent your interpretation of experiences you were going through at that time and what they meant about you. For example, if, as in the example above, your mother suffered from depression, she may not have been able to care for you or meet your needs as most mothers do. This may have led to you to conclude that it was your fault you couldn't get what you needed.

Now, it's time to identify your core beliefs. If they aren't immediately clear to you, don't worry. Sometimes it helps to picture another person in the experiences with you—a stranger or one of your friends—and imagine what this person would have felt or thought and how these experiences would have changed this person's life.

Uncovering Core Beliefs

To uncover your core beliefs, ask yourself the following questions:

* When you were experiencing this event—and coping with it to the best of your ability—what did you believe it meant about you that this was happening? (This is your interpretation of what happened to you.)

* What decisions did you make about your life or how you were going to live your life as a result of this event/experience?

* If this situation hadn't been in your life, how would your life be different?

Answers for the scenario outlined above might look like this:

* *I think I drew the conclusion that something was wrong with me because my mother didn't want to take care of me. Even though intellectually I now know this isn't true, as a child I felt that my needs weren't important, that having needs would make people not love me. So I tried not to let anyone know my needs.*

* *When I was little, I felt that I had to take care of myself because no one else was there to do it for me. I also decided that it was better to keep my needs and problems to myself, because when I didn't my mother couldn't handle them.*

* *If my mother hadn't been so depressed, I don't think I would be so independent, which has some value. But I also think I would be able to share myself more and have better relationships with friends and partners.*

Answer each of the three questions for your target experiences from the previous exercise. Then, using what you learn from these answers, articulate the core belief you developed as a result of these experiences. (You may also want to re-read your interpretations from the previous exercise to help you understand how being in the situation affected you before putting down your core belief.)

The two target experiences you identified in the previous exercise:

Target experience A: _____

Target experience B: _____

1. When you were experiencing this event—and coping with it to the best of your ability—what did you believe it meant about you that this was happening?

    Target experience A: _____

    Target experience B: _____

2. What decisions did you make about your life or how you were going to live your life as a result of this event/experience?

    Target experience A: _____

    Target experience B: _____

3. If this situation hadn't been in your life, how would your life be different?

    Target experience A: _____

    Target experience B: _____

Next, look over your answers. What core beliefs did you develop as a result of these experiences or events? For each experience, list your core beliefs and coping mechanisms in the following table.

Your Experience	Your Interpretation/Coping Mechanism	Core Belief
Example: *My mother was depressed.*	*My needs aren't important.* *I have to work hard for others to love me.*	*I have to be self-sufficient.* *I have to hide my true feelings/ needs.*

Now What Do You Do?

You have now successfully explored key life experiences and identified core beliefs you may not have previously recognized at a conscious level. You're probably beginning to think about the many different areas of your life affected by these core beliefs—and by others you haven't uncovered yet.

Next, we'll look at core beliefs related to your BED/CO and how they can keep you from reaching your goals for greater health and well-being. This will help you decide which beliefs you're ready to let go of, and which you aren't ready to change yet. There is no right or wrong choice here. You may find yourself afraid to let go of certain behaviors; even though they may have caused you some problems, these core beliefs are still familiar and comfortable to you. That's okay. It's neither possible nor advisable to change everything all at once. Permanent change requires small, determined steps that can be maintained. The next sections will help you start taking some of these small steps.

CORE BELIEFS AND YOUR BED/CO

First, how do your particular core beliefs affect your BED/CO? Work through the following exercise to explore the relationship between your core beliefs and your BED/CO.

Your Core Beliefs and Your BED/CO

Using the core beliefs you identified in the previous section, describe how you feel these beliefs affect your BED/CO.

Example:

Core belief: *I have to take care of myself because no one else will.*

Effect on your BED/CO: *This core belief makes it hard for me to ask for the help and support I need. Having to do everything on my own also creates more stress in my life, and when I am stressed I tend to binge more often.*

Core belief 1: _____

How this belief affects your BED/CO:

_____

_____

_____

Core belief 2: _____

How this belief affects your BED/CO:

_____

_____

_____
_____

How Your Core Beliefs Keep You Stuck in Your BED/CO

Unfortunately, you can't just wave a magic wand and have all of your problems disappear. (I'm saving that trick for another book.) However, a key start to making them disappear is to recognize how your beliefs keep you from reaching your goals. What do you think would happen if you stopped acting on these core beliefs?

This question may make you uncomfortable, even afraid. Why? Well, each of your core beliefs served an important purpose in your life at some point. As we've discussed throughout this section, your core beliefs developed to help you cope with difficult circumstances—to protect you and help you make it through bad times in your life.

As you saw in the previous exercise, your BED/CO behaviors often serve these core beliefs. Every behavior, no matter how much you may want to change it, serves some purpose. Let's look now at how your BED/CO behaviors both help and limit you.

The Pros and Cons of Your Core Beliefs

What are the pros and cons of keeping your core beliefs and the BED/CO behaviors associated with these core beliefs? To determine the pros of your core beliefs—and the BED/CO behaviors associated with them—ask yourself these questions:

1. What purpose do your behaviors or your size serve? (Example: _My bigger size makes me feel safe from attracting the opposite sex._)

    _____

    _____

2. In what ways are your behaviors effective strategies for coping with whatever is going on in your life? (Example: _Overeating takes my mind off my troubles. Bingeing helps me deal with my anger._)

    _____

    _____

3. Do you receive any special benefits from the behaviors associated with your BED/CO? (Example: *Comfort, relief of tension or anxiety, feeling nurtured.*)

_____

_____

4. What would be different in your life if these behaviors were no longer there? (Example: *I would have to be more responsible for taking care of my health and other areas in my life. Now, I can make excuses for not being responsible in my life because of my BED/CO.*)

_____

_____

5. Are there any aspects of your life that would get worse if you no longer had BED/CO? (Example: *I wouldn't get as much attention, because my family wouldn't worry about me as much. I might feel ignored or not as special.*)

_____

_____

To determine the cons of your core beliefs—and the BED/CO behaviors associated with them—ask yourself these questions:

1. If you weren't this size or didn't have BED/CO, what would you be doing with your life, career, relationships, etc. that you aren't doing now? (Example: *I'd ask my boss for a raise, get a different job, start dating.*)

_____

_____

2. How, specifically, do you feel your BED/CO and core beliefs hold you back? (Example: *I isolate myself and am not as sociable as I could be, and this affects my job performance.*)

_____

_____

3. How would your self-expression be different if you didn't have these core beliefs? (Example: *I would be more outgoing, I would dress in brighter colors.*)

_____

_____

You may find the preceding exercise more difficult than expected. You may be thinking, "I can't see *any* way in which my bingeing or overeating is good for me!" It's not unusual to feel this way. If you're having trouble seeing how these behaviors serve a purpose in your life, imagine that your best friend grew up in the same household as you did and has the same behaviors you do. Then ask yourself how these behaviors would have helped your friend cope.

Use the following table to list as many pros/advantages and cons/disadvantages of keeping your core beliefs as possible. Dig deep to see how holding onto these beliefs really affects the many different areas of your life.

Pros of Core Beliefs	Cons of Core Beliefs

Look over the pros and cons of your core beliefs. Which side has more validity for you today? Which side better supports your current goals for your life and your health? Now that you are aware of both how your core beliefs once served you and how they are currently keeping you stuck in your BED/ CO, you have the opportunity to choose what you want to do about these beliefs.

Deciding What to Do About Your Old Core Beliefs

Congratulations! You have identified your core beliefs, explored how they relate to your BED/CO, and learned how these old beliefs keep you stuck. You are now more aware of these beliefs and their effects on your life. Even if you go no further right now, you will have accomplished something that will help you eventually reach your goals. The next step is deciding what you want to do about these old beliefs.

HOW READY ARE YOU TO CHANGE?

Before you prepare to make any kind of significant change, it is important to assess your level of readiness. Rate your readiness to change your core beliefs on a scale of 1–10, with 1 being "no way do I want to change anything" and 10 being "sign me up—I'm ready to go for it." Whatever number you choose, be honest with yourself about where you are today in terms of your readiness to change.

Are you ready to change your core beliefs?

1	2	3	4	5	6	7	8	9	10

Based on your level of readiness, you can now choose which core beliefs you want to hold onto and which you want to let go.

You chose a readiness to change of 1–5. If you rated your readiness for change as between 1 and 5, you may want to review the pros and cons list to see if you can find at least one reason why change is worth working toward. At these levels of readiness, you may want to change but not believe that change is possible. Change takes willingness—sometimes we block this willingness with a "yes, but" statement that keeps us from making any forward progress.

"Yes, But" Statements

Make a list of your "yes, but" statements in the following table. These are the thoughts that immediately spring to mind when you think about challenging your core beliefs. Next to each "yes, but" statement, put an argument for the defense: Imagine you're in a court of law and the prosecution has just presented evidence against your ability to change. Step over to the defense table and argue on your own behalf, offering evidence in support of your ability to change.

Prosecution's Argument: *I'd like to change my core beliefs, but...*	Defense's Argument:
Example: *When I was 21, I tried to become more independent and not such a caretaker but it didn't work out, so why bother now?*	*When I tried making changes before I was younger and less mature. I have more support in my life now and I can see how not making a change has negatively impacted my life.*

Now that you've completed the preceding exercise, has your readiness to change altered? Circle the number that best applies to you:

Are you ready to make change your core beliefs?

1	2	3	4	5	6	7	8	9	10

If you still don't feel ready to change (you chose 5 or less), don't beat yourself up or try to force the issue. Rather, bookmark this page and read on; you can return to this chapter at a later time. Also, consider using an affirmation such as "I am working toward being ready for change in my life." Whenever you feel down on yourself for not having changed, say this affirmation to remind yourself that you are still in the game, you're just making your changes slowly.

If your readiness for change went up (above 5), proceed to the next section.

You chose a readiness for change of 6–10. If you rated your readiness for change at 6 or above, you may have some doubts about your ability to change but are willing to give it a try. You've probably already discovered resources that can help you get past your doubts, so that you continue to move toward your goals. These resources may include specific skills or techniques, people, or other forms of support.

Resources and Skills

List the resources and skills at your disposal; write down anything that can support you in making the changes you've committed to: (Use your journal to list additional resources and skills.)

Example: *My faith has gotten me through a lot of hard times.*

Example: *When I have a hard time doing something, I just say to myself over and over "You can do it, you can do it." It's like I'm being a cheerleader for myself!*

Example: *My wife is my best support system. She helps me see the big picture.*

1. _____

_____

2. _____

_____

3. _____

_____

Excellent! You're now ready to change core beliefs that are unhealthy and keep you stuck in your BED/CO. However, change does not happen overnight. Look at this process as a long-term one and be gentle with yourself whenever you feel your core beliefs aren't changing fast enough.

Letting Go of Unhealthy Core Beliefs

You've set your intention to change your core beliefs and are ready to take action. The next step is to decide which core beliefs you want to change, and then develop a system of signals to alert you whenever you fall back on the old core beliefs.

DECIDING WHICH CORE BELIEFS TO RELEASE

As we discussed earlier in the chapter, even an unhealthy core belief such as "I have to do everything for myself" has some value. This type of core belief can make you very productive at work—everyone will know they can rely on you to get the job done. Why give up such a belief?

Consider letting go of such a belief—or modifying it—when its cost outweighs its benefits. Check whether the core belief is in alignment with your goals for your health and well-being, including your desire to overcome your BED or CO. It can be easier to let go of a core belief when you recognize that it is holding you back from asking for help with your BED or CO—and from living the life you want.

Getting Motivated to Change

Start by listing core beliefs you want to change; these may include the target core beliefs you've used in previous exercises. (Use your journal to work on additional core beliefs.) Next to each core belief, record any strong motivating factors that will help you remember why you want to change this belief.

Core Belief You Want to Change	What Motivates You to Change This Belief
Example: *I have to take care of myself because no one else will.*	*I don't want my children to grow up feeling that they have to do the same thing they see me doing.* *I want to have the time and energy to go back to school. I can't if I'm always so overwhelmed and stressed out.*

Once you've filled in this table, make several copies of it. Put these in strategic places to remind yourself of your motivation to change. Put a copy on your refrigerator, on your bathroom mirror, in your car, on your desk—anywhere you will see it on a daily basis. Regularly reminding yourself why you are changing will make the process easier.

HOW WILL YOU KNOW YOU ARE CHANGING?

Life is very busy and chaotic. As a result, sometimes keeping your goals on track can seem overwhelming. You may be thinking, "Oh, great! Now I have something else I have to do." Whenever your goal is to change something about yourself, it's a good idea to give yourself as much help as possible. One way to do this is to create simple systems to prop you up as you're going through these changes. The following system will help you identify red flags that indicate you're living or acting from your old core beliefs.

Looking for Red Flags: Staying Aware of Your Patterns

It's important to know, without a shadow of a doubt, when you are acting from your unhealthy core beliefs. What emotions and physical sensations are associated with your old patterns? Are specific body postures associated with these core beliefs? Are they linked to a certain way you dress, or a type of person you hang out with? List the many ways—both subtle and obvious—that these old core beliefs are integrated into your life. Be creative—think of yourself as a character in a play and describe what you learn from watching this character. (Your observations may include different categories than those in the following example.)

Example:

Core belief you're letting go of: *Feeling like I have to hide my feelings/that I can't show people the real me.*

Emotions:	*Anger and frustration.*
Physical sensations:	*Tightness in my upper chest and the back of my neck.*
Thoughts:	*No one wants to hear what I have to say; what I'm feeling isn't important.*
People:	*When I feel like this, I tend to avoid my mother because she has always told me to not let other people see me cry.*
Foods and cravings:	*When I feel this way, I tend to binge on salty chips.*
BED/CO behaviors:	*Bingeing, isolating myself.*
Posture associated: with this belief:	*Rigid, tight.*
Places:	*I often go to bars when I feel this way to drink, eat, and hide out.*
How old do you feel when in this belief?	*Very young, like 8 years old.*

1. Core belief you're letting go of: _____

Posture associated with this belief: _____

Emotions: _____

Physical sensations: _____

Thoughts: _____

People: _____

Places: _____

How old do you feel when in this belief? _____

Foods and cravings: _____

BED/CO behaviors: _____

Other ways this core belief shows up in your life:

_____

_____

_____

_____

2. Core belief you're letting go of: _____

   Posture associated with this belief: _____

   Emotions: _____

   Physical sensations: _____

   Thoughts: _____

   People: _____

   Places: _____

   How old do you feel when in this belief? _____

   Foods and cravings: _____

   BED/CO behaviors: _____

   Other ways this core belief shows up in your life:

   _____

   _____

   _____

   _____

You may find that one core belief has similar body postures, emotions, and so on, as another. Sometimes core beliefs can overlap—perhaps because they came into being during the same period of your life, or are related to a common experience. If this is the case, feel free to combine them and work on them together. Otherwise, choose one to work on first, focusing your efforts on it for an extended period of time. Then come back to the other core beliefs you want to change. Don't try to take on too much at one time. Choose realistic goals, goals you can accomplish.

CREATING YOUR GUIDING PRINCIPLES

As you let go of old core beliefs, there will be a vacuum where the old beliefs once were. At the beginning of this chapter, we talked about Tony, one of whose core beliefs was "bigger is better." For Tony, the part of him that had been bullied by his older brother—his child self—felt safer and more at ease when he was bigger. How could he feel safe without that old core belief? By filling that vacuum with new, healthy guiding principles.

The process of letting go involves a number of phases: understanding how and why your core beliefs developed; acknowledging the pros and cons of these beliefs; assessing your readiness to change; and recognizing your current resources and skills. Now that you've used the exercises of this chapter to let go of some of your old core beliefs, you have a vacuum where those beliefs once were—a vacuum just waiting to be filled with new guiding principles.

Unlike core beliefs, guiding principles are under your creative control. Where core beliefs were coping strategies from the past, guiding principles are instead conscious decisions about how you want to live your life. Are you ready to embrace new guiding principles aligned with recovering from BED/CO? This is exactly what you will be working on in the next exercise.

Imagine!

Find a comfortable place where you will not be disturbed. Sit, don't lie flat—you may want to prop your feet on a footstool. Listen to some soothing music if you like. Keep your eyes closed—or, if you don't feel comfortable doing so, focus on something pleasant in your surroundings, such as a flower or a favorite painting. Once you're settled, you will begin to imagine your life with a new set of guiding principles.

First, imagine what it would be like to take the old core beliefs and give them a proper burial. Imagine yourself wrapping the old beliefs in a blanket or putting them in a box, and then taking them to a place you like outside, perhaps under a big tree or in a garden. Next, imagine yourself digging a hole in the soft earth and placing the package or box into this hole. After you've covered up the hole, thank these old beliefs for helping you get this far in your life. Thank them for providing comfort and safety to you in the past. Say goodbye and offer them any blessings you'd like.

Next, imagine leaving this area to go to a place where you feel very safe. This could be a favorite beach, a park bench, or somewhere inside your house. Notice how it feels to be there without the old core beliefs. Notice any emotions you feel, any thoughts that come to mind. Imagine a whole day in your life without these core beliefs. Who are you with? What are you doing? Where do you go? What do you eat? What types of foods appeal to you? How do you feel about your body?

Now, consider what guiding principles you want to have fill the vacuum left by the old beliefs. Choose principles that will help you in some of the ways the old beliefs did. Your old beliefs may have served as your anchor during a period of turbulence in your life. Your new beliefs should serve as an anchor in the new life you're creating through recovery. New beliefs should help you stay motivated, keep you on track, and be important enough to you that they can replace old beliefs. For example, an old core belief may have helped you deal with feeling helpless or vulnerable as a child because you didn't have many resources. At the time, you couldn't do much more than what you did to take care of yourself. Now, recognizing that you are an adult and have other options, you may want to focus your attention on other ways to take care of yourself. Spend a little time daydreaming about what new guiding principles you want to embrace; then, when you are finished, record your thoughts below:

_____

_____

_____

_____

_____

_____

List your new guiding principles:

Old Core Belief	New Guiding Principle
Example: *Bigger is better.*	*Exercising helps me feel strong and able to take care of myself.*

Don't underestimate the ability of your mind to influence your body and even your spirit. The mind-body connection is very powerful indeed—and underused. You can do this exercise many times; each time you will learn something new about yourself. Consider recording your imaginings so that you can replay them occasionally for yourself.

═══

Supporting Healthy Core Beliefs

A new guiding principle can be a fragile thing. A new guiding principle is much like a baby, entirely dependent on her parents. You are the parent, and you must nurture your new principles, allowing them time to get stronger and bigger and more deeply ingrained. If you embrace a new guiding principle, but then neglect it, forgetting about it rather than consciously supporting it, the principle will grow weak.

Use the skills and resources you identified earlier in this chapter to support your healthy principles. You can also create affirmations to counter any negative self-talk you experience when trying to live from your new principles. *Affirmations* are positive statements that you say to yourself to remind you of your goals and prevent yourself from getting sidetracked.

For each new guiding principle, answer the questions in the following exercise.

Supporting Your New Core Beliefs

Your new guiding principle: _____, can be supported by:

(Example: *"Healthier is better" can be supported by 1) continuing to work on my recovery from BED/CO, and 2) soothing my anxiety with self-care, such as by getting a massage or taking a walk with my dog when I feel anxious.*)

_____

_____

_____

Who in your life will support your new core beliefs and how?

(Example: *My friend at work has offered to walk with me at lunchtime; my wife helps me by cooking healthy meals at home.*)

_____

_____

_____

What affirmations will you use if you get discouraged or find yourself engaging in negative self-talk?

(Example: *Being mindful of my health brings me great peace and safety.*)

_____

_____

_____

SUMMARY

Challenging core beliefs isn't easy. However, by completing the exercises of this chapter, you've taken an important step toward clearing your mind of old beliefs that aren't consistent with your recovery goals. You are no longer at the mercy of beliefs that had become unconscious and automatic. Instead, you are committed to letting go of unhealthy beliefs, and have created new guiding principles that will support you in your journey to recovery.

CHAPTER 9

Co-occurring Diagnoses

written with Andrew Stropko, Ph.D.

Eating disorders are often accompanied by certain other disorders; these include depression, anxiety, and personality disorders. These co-occurring disorders may be related to malnutrition or undernutrition or substance use disorders, or may have existed prior to your diagnosis with BED/CO. Treating co-occurring disorders is key to recovery from BED/CO; if left untreated, these disorders can trigger behaviors associated with BED/CO.

DEPRESSION AND ANXIETY

After the common cold, depression and anxiety are the most prevalent illnesses known to humankind. When most of us think of depression, we think of feelings of sadness. However, symptoms of more severe forms of depression include loss of interest in previously enjoyed pastimes, sleep disturbance, feelings of guilt, appetite disturbance, not feeling good about yourself, fatigue, headaches, diminished concentration, clouded thinking, and thoughts of self-harm, among others.

Although anxiety is a little less familiar to us, its severe form is well-known, and commonly referred to as a nervous breakdown. Anxiety is marked by tension, worry, a preoccupation with problems, an inability to relax, fear, apprehension, and a sense of impending doom. A myriad of physical symptoms often accompany these characteristics of anxiety, including difficulty breathing, feeling faint, excessive perspiration, muscle tension, increased heart rate, and stomach disturbances.

BED/CO and Depression

Many people with BED/CO report that their bingeing or overeating is triggered by feelings of depression or anxiety. Others, although unable to identify specific precursors, nonetheless report that overeating diminishes a tension that is hard to define.

People with BED are more likely to develop bipolar disorder (also known as manic depression), anxiety disorders, bulimia, and substance use disorders at some time in their lives than those without BED (Javaras et al. 2008). Depression may explain why compulsive overeaters and those with BED eat in response to low moods and have difficulty controlling their eating (Masheb and Grilo 2006). Women with BED who are very obese (who have a BMI over 40 kg/m²) are at higher risk for experiencing significant problems with depression; this may be a motivating factor in seeking treatment (Fabricatore and Wadden 2003). In addition, researchers studying the family history of binge eaters have found that close female relatives are more likely to experience depression or anxiety, to have a substance use disorder, or to suffer from anorexia or BED—pointing to a possible common mechanism for familial transmission of these co-occurring disorders (Lilenfeld et al. 2008).

Obese individuals are more likely to have mood and anxiety disorders (up to two times that of non-obese individuals), alcohol use disorders, and personality disorders than those who are of normal weight. Being only moderately overweight was also associated with an increased risk for anxiety and substance use disorders (Petry et al. 2007).

For people with BED/CO, in addition to the characteristics of depression listed previously, depression is likely to manifest through the following cycles:

* Poor self-esteem—thinking poorly of yourself, nurturing yourself with food, then blaming yourself because of weight gain.

* Guilt related to a lack of self-control—overeating, feeling guilty because you can't stop yourself, then overeating to medicate the unpleasantness of the guilt.

* Emotional dysregulation—being emotionally out of control, overeating due to emotional distress, then suffering guilt about bingeing or overeating.

The following self-test (Zung 1965) will help you assess whether or not you are depressed. If you are depressed, use your answers to the test as a foundation for talking to your health care provider.

Zung Self-Rating Depression Scale

For each item, circle the response that most closely represents your feelings and behaviors. Add all of the circled responses together for your total: (Since items 5 and 7 have to do with food and weight, if you are on a diet, answer these two items from the standpoint of what your answers would be if you were not on the diet.)

1. I feel downhearted and blue

    1 A little of the time   2 Some of the time   3 A good part of the time   4 Most of the time

2. Morning is when I feel the best

    4 A little of the time   3 Some of the time   2 A good part of the time   1 Most of the time

3. I have crying spells or feel like it

    1 A little of the time   2 Some of the time   3 A good part of the time   4 Most of the time

4. I have trouble sleeping at night

    1 A little of the time   2 Some of the time   3 A good part of the time   4 Most of the time

5. I eat as much as I used to

    4 A little of the time   3 Some of the time   2 A good part of the time   4 Most of the time

6. I still enjoy sex

    4 A little of the time   3 Some of the time   2 A good part of the time   1 Most of the time

7. I notice that I am losing weight

    1 A little of the time   2 Some of the time   3 A good part of the time   4 Most of the time

8. I have trouble with constipation

    1 A little of the time   2 Some of the time   3 A good part of the time   4 Most of the time

9. My heart beats faster than usual

    1 A little of the time   2 Some of the time   3 A good part of the time   4 Most of the time

10. I get tired for no reason

    1 A little of the time   2 Some of the time   3 A good part of the time   4 Most of the time

11. My mind is as clear as it used to be

    4 A little of the time   3 Some of the time   2 A good part of the time   1 Most of the time

12. I find it easy to do the things I used to

    4 A little of the time   3 Some of the time   2 A good part of the time   1 Most of the time

13. I am restless and can't keep still

    1 A little of the time   2 Some of the time   3 A good part of the time   4 Most of the time

14. I feel hopeful about the future

    4 A little of the time   3 Some of the time   2 A good part of the time   1 Most of the time

15. I am more irritable than usual

    1 A little of the time   2 Some of the time   3 A good part of the time   4 Most of the time

16. I find it easy to make decisions

    4 A little of the time   3 Some of the time   2 A good part of the time   1 Most of the time

17. I feel that I am useful and needed

    4 A little of the time   3 Some of the time   2 A good part of the time   1 Most of the time

18. My life is pretty full

    4 A little of the time   3 Some of the time   2 A good part of the time   1 Most of the time

19. I feel that others would be better off if I were dead

    1 A little of the time   2 Some of the time   3 A good part of the time   4 Most of the time

20. I still enjoy the things I used to do

    4 A little of the time   3 Some of the time   2 A good part of the time   1 Most of the time

Although the Zung Self-Rating Depression Scale does not diagnose, it does offer an idea of the severity of depression symptoms. A total score of 39 or less suggests no significant depression; 40 to 47 suggests minimal to mild depression; 48 to 55 suggests moderate to marked depression; and 56 or greater suggests severe to extreme depression.

Anxiety and BED/CO

Anxiety and BED/CO can be a vicious circle. Researchers have found that 71 percent of those with BED also experience significant anxiety (Castellini et al. 2008). Whether or not diagnosed with BED, obese individuals are at higher risk for generalized anxiety disorder, panic attacks, and depression. For people with BED/CO, in addition to the symptoms of anxiety previously discussed, anxiety often manifests as the following:

*   Social discomfort—discomfort in social situations due to body dissatisfaction and a fear of being judged for being overweight or obese.

*   Trust issues—not feeling safe with others; a fear of being hurt.

*   Maturity fears—feeling unready or ill-equipped to handle the demands or expectations of adulthood. Individuals with BED/CO who are overweight tend to have more maturity fears than normal-weight individuals (Tuthill et al. 2006).

These various manifestations of anxiety can trigger bingeing and overeating. The following self-test (Zung 1971) will help you assess what level of anxiety you presently have.

Zung Self-Rating Anxiety Scale

For each item, circle the response that most closely represents your feelings and behaviors. Add all of the circled responses together for your total:

1. I feel more nervous and anxious than usual

    1 A little of the time   2 Some of the time   3 A good part of the time   4 Most of the time

2. I feel afraid for no reason at all

    1 A little of the time   2 Some of the time   3 A good part of the time   4 Most of the time

3. I get upset easily or feel panicky

    1 A little of the time   2 Some of the time   3 A good part of the time   4 Most of the time

4. I feel like I am falling apart and falling to pieces

    1 A little of the time   2 Some of the time   3 A good part of the time   4 Most of the time

5. I feel that everything is all right and nothing bad will happen

    4 A little of the time   3 Some of the time   2 A good part of the time   1 Most of the time

6. My arms and legs shake and tremble

    1 A little of the time   2 Some of the time   3 A good part of the time   4 Most of the time

7. I am bothered by headaches and neck and back pain

    1 A little of the time   2 Some of the time   3 A good part of the time   4 Most of the time

8. I feel weak and get tired easily

    1 A little of the time   2 Some of the time   3 A good part of the time   4 Most of the time

9. I feel calm and can sit still easily

    4 A little of the time   3 Some of the time   2 A good part of the time   1 Most of the time

10. I can feel my heart beating fast

    1 A little of the time   2 Some of the time   3 A good part of the time   4 Most of the time

11. I am bothered by dizzy spells

    1 A little of the time   2 Some of the time   3 A good part of the time   4 Most of the time

12. I have fainting spells or feel faint

    1 A little of the time   2 Some of the time   3 A good part of the time   4 Most of the time

13. I can breath in and out easily

    4 A little of the time   3 Some of the time   2 A good part of the time   1 Most of the time

14. I get feelings of numbness and tingling in my fingers and toes

    1 A little of the time   2 Some of the time   3 A good part of the time   4 Most of the time

15. I am bothered by stomachaches or indigestion

    1 A little of the time   2 Some of the time   3 A good part of the time   4 Most of the time

16. I have to empty my bladder often

    1 A little of the time   2 Some of the time   3 A good part of the time   4 Most of the time

17. My hands are usually dry and warm

    4 A little of the time   3 Some of the time   2 A good part of the time   1 Most of the time

18. My face gets hot and blushes

    1 A little of the time   2 Some of the time   3 A good part of the time   4 Most of the time

19. I fall asleep easily and get a good night's rest

    4 A little of the time   3 Some of the time   2 A good part of the time   1 Most of the time

20. I have nightmares

    1 A little of the time   2 Some of the time   3 A good part of the time   4 Most of the time

A total score of 35 or less suggests no significant anxiety; 36 to 47 suggests minimal to moderate anxiety; 48 to 59 suggests marked to severe anxiety; and 60 or greater suggests extreme anxiety. However, only a healthcare professional can diagnose an anxiety disorder; if your anxiety score is high, talk to your healthcare professional about it.

Fortunately, there are many ways to treat depression and anxiety. We'll discuss some of these treatment options later in this chapter.

PERSONALITY DISORDERS

Personality disorders are caused by problematic personality traits that have usually been present since you were very young. The problems these traits create tend to show up in all the spheres of your life. Just as depression and anxiety are psychiatric diagnoses, so are personality disorders.

For several reasons, personality disorders that typically occur with BED and CO are often neglected in comparison to mood disorders. First, professionals tend to be more focused on major psychiatric conditions, such as depression and anxiety. Second, an individual's health insurance many not cover treatment for personality disorders, whereas it usually will cover mood disorders. Third, personality disorders are less obvious and thus harder to diagnose than mood disorders.

There are many different personality disorders. Interestingly, some personality disorders are more common in people with BED or CO, while others are more common in people with bulimia or anorexia. The most common personality disorders in people with BED are avoidant personality disorder, obsessive-compulsive personality disorder (Picot and Lilenfeld 2003), histrionic personality disorder, and borderline personality disorder (Specker et al. 1994). Similarly, avoidant, dependent, and obsessive-compulsive personality disorders may occur in people with CO (Mauri et al. 2008). Antisocial personality disorder is prevalent in both BED and CO (Johnson et al. 2006). Let's explore in greater detail the different personality disorders most frequently found in people with BED/CO.

Avoidant Personality Disorder

Individuals with *avoidant personality disorder* are anxious and withdrawn, and may feel inadequate in social situations. People with an avoidant personality sometimes feel like wallflowers who want to get involved but don't have the social skills or feel too anxious to do so. They are also overly sensitive to criticism and have trouble becoming involved with others unless they are sure they are liked. They often worry about being rejected or criticized. They may have difficulty facing their problems, choosing instead to turn a blind eye.

Dependent Personality Disorder

Individuals with *dependent personality disorder* need a great deal of support and nurturance, have difficulty making decisions without advice, and often go to great lengths to feel accepted—including taking on unpleasant tasks they don't really want to do. Individuals with a dependent personality are people pleasers; they often have low self-esteem and may feel guilty, worry excessively, and be very self-critical.

Obsessive-Compulsive Personality Disorder (OCPD)

Individuals with *obsessive-compulsive personality disorder* (OCPD) are excessively preoccupied with organization, perfectionism, and control. As a result, people with OCPD love lists, schedules, rules, and regulations. At times perfectionists to a fault, they tend toward work addiction, emphasizing a dedication to getting things done and neglecting avocational enjoyment. People with OCPD can be stiff shirts who don't seem to be having much fun, in part because they feel they have to do everything themselves because others won't do it the "right way." For people with OCPD, everything has a place and there is a place for everything.

Histrionic Personality Disorder (HPD)

Individuals with *histrionic personality disorder* (HPD) have a strong need for attention and are emotionally expressive. Others often see people with HPD as drama queens (or kings). Individuals with a histrionic personality type sometimes perceive relationships as more intimate than they really are—and, like a Pollyanna, report everything as great even in the midst of chaos or dysfunction. People with HPD often have trouble acknowledging unpleasantness.

Antisocial Personality Disorder (APD)

Individuals with antisocial personality disorder (APD) tend to violate societal norms, doing things quickly without consideration of the consequences. They may lack remorse after lying, stealing, or hurting someone. Others often see people with APD as rebels or as having a chip on the shoulder—either way, as someone who constantly gets into power struggles with authority figures.

Borderline Personality Disorder (BPD)

Individuals with *borderline personality disorder* (BPD) have a high degree of impulsivity and display a pattern of instability in interpersonal relationships and mood. They often have difficulty understanding themselves and look at interpersonal relationships as black and white, either putting others on a pedestal or assuming the worst. People with BPD may feel emotions more intensely than others and experience intense mood swings. Finally, people with BPD tend to lack focus and purpose. They appear to need chaos to thrive.

Each of these personality types has a prominent need. Individuals with avoidant personalities want to feel included, to be part of the group. Dependent individuals need nurturance. Individuals with obsessive-compulsive personality disorder have a strong desire for control and order. Those with histrionic personalities need attention—which explains their flair or penchant for creating drama: they need to be center stage. Those with antisocial personalities need to assert their independence and not be controlled by social conventions; when stressed, they tend to act out or rebel. Those with borderline personality disorder tend to seek out chaos, perhaps because their younger lives were full of chaos and this is what makes them feel in their comfort zone.

When this need is not met, a person with BED/CO may use food to satisfy the uncomfortable feelings associated with the unmet need. For example, an individual with dependent personality disorder may work very hard and sacrifice a great deal of time and energy to please her supervisor. However, if the supervisor doesn't notice the worker's effort to gain support and nurturance, the dependent individual may soothe her resultant frustration by overeating.

TREATMENT OPTIONS

A variety of conventional and alternative approaches are used to treat depression, anxiety, and personality disorders; these include medication, exercise, dietary supplements, acupuncture, and massage, among others.

Medication for Depression and Anxiety in Those with BED/CO

Several medications have been proposed to reduce weight and treat depression in binge eating disorder. (Because most of the research on these medications has been short term, no conclusions about the longer-term effects of the medication can be drawn yet.) Researchers who looked at fourteen studies on medication for treatment of BED found that medications may aid individuals in stopping binge eating in the short term (twelve to sixteen weeks), but that symptoms usually reoccur once medications are discontinued. Two medications that were studied—topiramate (a prescription medication sold under the name Topamax) and orlistat (the weight loss drug marketed as Xenical or alli)—enhanced the weight loss achieved with behavioral therapies (Reas and Grilo 2008).

Because many people with BED/CO also have depression, antidepressants are often used in the treatment of BED/CO. The antidepressant Luvox decreases the frequency of binge episodes and can lead to weight loss; higher doses of Luvox than typically prescribed for depression were more effective (60 milligrams/day). Other antidepressants, such as Zoloft, Prozac, and Celexa—all of which are in the same class, known as selective serotonin reuptake inhibitors (SSRIs)—were also found to decrease bingeing (Appolinario and McElroy 2004). Side effects of SSRIs include dry mouth, sedation, stomach upset, and sexual side effects (inability to ejaculate, difficulty achieving orgasm). In addition, buproprion (Wellbutrin), an atypical antidepressant that is not an SSRI, can produce significant weight loss; however, Wellbutrin is not approved specifically for weight loss (Gadde, Krishnan, and Drezner 1997). Side effects of Wellbutrin include dry mouth, stomach upset, constipation, muscle aches, and loss of appetite.

Topiramate (Topamax), an antiseizure medication also used to treat bipolar disorders, can decrease bingeing behavior, improve depression, and cause weight loss in individuals with BED (McElroy et al. 2007). Side effects include dizziness, insomnia, depression, nausea, difficulty with concentration, and attention and memory problems.

The association between BED/CO and obesity has also prompted the study of sibutramine (Meridia), an appetite suppressant. Meridia has been found to significantly reduce depression symptoms, weight, and bingeing (Appolinario et al. 2002). Common side effects include dry mouth, insomnia, constipation, increased blood pressure and heart rate, and headaches.

Exercise

Many studies support the efficacy of exercise in treating anxiety and depression. Both physical activity and exercise have a beneficial effect on mild to moderate depression and anxiety (Paluska and Schwenk 2000). In fact, exercise may be equal to medication in treating depression, more effective in reducing recurrence of depression than medication alone (Babyak et al. 2000), and as effective as psychotherapy (Greist et al. 1978)—even in patients with the most severe depression.

Herbs and Dietary Supplements

Herbs have been used for hundreds of years to treat depression and anxiety. Because many herbs work in a similar way to prescription medications, if you are taking prescription antidepressants, be sure to speak with your health care professional prior to taking any over-the-counter herbal products. There is little research so far on the use of these supplements on those with BED/CO who also have depression/anxiety.

S-ADENOSYLMETHIONINE

S-adenosylmethionine (SAMe) is a naturally occurring substance in the body involved in the production of serotonin (the brain chemical affected by most common prescription antidepressants). People suffering from depression may have lower levels of natural s-adenosylmethionine. Several smaller, short-term studies have found SAMe supplements as effective as some prescription antidepressants (imipramine), but with less significant side effects (Delle, Pancheri, and Scapicchio 2002; Rosenbaum et al. 2007).

ST. JOHN'S WORT

St. John's wort is a traditional herb used to treat depression. Researchers have found St. John's wort to be better than placebos and equal to prescription antidepressants in treating mild to moderate depression, with fewer side effects (Linde, Berner, and Kriston 2008). St. John's wort may also be effective in treating obsessive-compulsive disorder (Taylor and Kobak 2000) and generalized anxiety disorder (Davidson and Connor 2001).

VALERIAN

Traditionally, valerian root has been used to treat insomnia; research has found that it significantly improves sleep quality (Donath et al. 2000). Valerian is also effective for reducing situational anxiety (Kohnen and Oswald1988) and stress-related insomnia (Wheatley 2001). In addition, valerian may also be useful in treating generalized anxiety disorder; one study found it equal to the prescription medication Valium, however neither was better than a placebo (Andreatini et al. 2002).

5-HYDROXYTRYPTOPHAN

Tryptophan is an amino acid that occurs in milk and other foods. In the body, it is converted into 5-Hydroxytryptophan (5-HTP), which then crosses into the brain to become serotonin. Supplementation with 5-HTP can improve symptoms of depression (Shaw, Turner, and Del Mar 2002). In fact, 5-HTP may be as effective as some prescription antidepressants (Luvox and Tofranil) (Poldinger, Calanchini, and Schwatz 1991).

5-HTP may also reduce symptoms of anxiety (Kahn and Westenburg 1985), decrease appetite, and help with weight loss (Cangiano et al. 1992). Furthermore, 5-HTP may reduce anxiety in those with anxiety disorders without depression (Kahn, Westenburg, and Verhoven 1987) and may prevent panic attacks (Schruers, Pols, and Overbeek 2002). Finally, 5-HTP can be taken at bedtime to help with insomnia.

L-tryptophan—a precursor to 5-HTP supplements—was taken off the market in 1989 after being associated with a syndrome called eosinophilia-myalgia syndrome (EMS), which was later thought due to a contaminant from a single manufacturer. There have been no recently reported cases of EMS associated with 5-HTP.

Herbs and Dietary Supplements for Depression and Anxiety

Herb	Dose	Side effects	Cautions
S-adenosyl-methionine (SAMe)	Start with 200 milligrams twice daily; increase as needed, to a maximum of 800 milligrams twice a day. Use products that are packaged in blister packs to avoid a breakdown of ingredients.	May cause insomnia, anxiety, and excitation.	Those with a history of bipolar disease should not take SAMe, except under supervision of their health care professional, as it may trigger mania.
St. John's wort	Start with 300 milligrams, three times daily; increase as needed, to a maximum of 1200 milligrams per day. (St. John's wort is standardized to a 3.0-percent hyperforin content.)	May increase photosensitivity, leading to sunburn, so prolonged sun exposure should be avoided.	Those with a history of bipolar disease should not take St. John's wort except under supervision of their health care professional, as it may trigger mania. If you are on birth control pills, medication for HIV, or antibiotics, consult your doctor before taking St. John's wort.
Valerian	300 milligrams two or three times a day for anxiety. Take 900 milligrams at bedtime to aid sleep.	May cause headaches, upset stomach, dizziness, and low body temperature.	Should not be used during pregnancy or while breastfeeding. If you are on a prescription antidepressant, consult your doctor before taking, as it may interact with some antidepressant medications. Do not take with medications that are sedating or while driving.

5- HTP	50–300 milligrams per day.	May cause heartburn, stomachaches, nausea, and diarrhea.	Persons with bipolar disorder should not take 5-HTP except under supervision of their health care professional, as it may trigger mania. If you are on a prescription antidepressant, consult your doctor before taking, as it may interact with some antidepressant medications.

OTHER SUPPLEMENTS

In chapter 3 we discussed B vitamins and omega-3 fatty acids in detail. These supplements also have a special importance in treating mood disorders. B vitamins—and particularly folic acid—have been shown to improve the effectiveness of antidepressant medications (Taylor et al. 2003; Coppen and Bailey 2000). People suffering from depression tend to be deficient in omega-3 fatty acids; research has found supplementation with omega-3 fatty acids effective in treating depression. As well, in individuals with severe depression, higher levels of omega-3 fatty acids are associated with decreased suicide risk (Sublette et al. 2006). If you have been diagnosed with depression, whether or not you are on prescription medications, you should take a B-complex vitamin and omega-3 fatty acids on a daily basis. (For dosages, refer to chapter 3.) Finally, research has found that people with borderline personality disorder who take omega-3 fatty acids have fewer symptoms of aggression and anger (Zanarini and Frankenburt 2003).

Acupuncture

Acupuncture originated in China more than three thousand years ago. It involves the placement of thin needles along energy channels in the body, and may help depression by stimulating the release of the brain chemicals norepinephrine and serotonin (Han 1986). Research on acupuncture for depression offers conflicting results. However, some research has found acupuncture as effective as certain antidepressant medications (Smith and Hay 2005). Individuals with anxiety who were treated with acupuncture in addition to behavioral desensitization showed significantly higher cure rates than those treated with either therapy alone (Guizhen et al. 1998). Acupuncture can also be effective in treating post-traumatic stress disorder (Hollifield et al. 2007).

Massage Therapy

Massage is not just for relaxation. Massage can be effective in treating depression (Field et al. 1992) through its impact on brain waves (it shifts them to a pattern associated with happy feelings) (Jones and Field 1999) and the relaxation it produces. When used to treat children with post-traumatic stress disorder, massage was found to reduce anxiety (Field et al. 1996). Massage is also associated with improved symptoms in individuals with eating disorders, depression, and physical illness (Hart 2001; Field, Martinez, and Nawrock 1998). The use of essential oils (aromatherapy) in addition to massage therapy may also help treat depression and anxiety. Relevant essential oils include bergamot, geranium, German chamomile, lavender, and rosemary (Zand 1999).

Other Therapies

Other approaches to treating depression and anxiety include yoga, music therapy, pet therapy, reading, and relaxation therapy. Yoga breathing techniques, when practiced for thirty minutes every day for thirty days, accelerated improvement in patients with depression (Janakiramaiah et al. 2000). A review of studies on music therapy, showed it to be effective in reducing symptoms of depression (Jones and Feld 1999; Maratos et al. 2008).

Although most effective in treating anxiety, relaxation therapy is also used to treat depression. Relaxation therapy includes any technique that enables the individual to voluntarily relax; examples include meditation, breath work, guided imagery, and progressive muscle relaxation. Research has found relaxation therapy equal to cognitive behavioral therapy (Reynolds and Coats 1986; Murphy et al. 1995) and some antidepressant medications (Murphy et al. 1995). Relaxation therapy combined with medication produces better results than medication alone (Bowers 1990).

SUMMARY

Depression, anxiety, and personality disorders commonly occur with BED/CO. Fortunately, there are many ways to treat these conditions. The use of complementary and alternative therapies, exercise, and dietary supplements can decrease symptoms and may enhance the efficacy of medication.

PART 3

Healing the Spirit

CHAPTER 10

Coping with Stress

Stress is a fact of modern life that cannot be eliminated. Stress comes from how we perceive events. These perceptions are different for different people. Similarly, we have individual ways of coping with stress. Stress affects both our health and our mood, and can contribute to the development of unhealthy eating patterns. In this chapter, we'll focus on the physical effects of stress and its connection to eating disorders. Then, in chapter 11, we'll explore tools for managing stress.

THE BASICS OF STRESS

Whether you're a caveman or woman being chased by a tiger or you're a modern human who works a full-time job, goes to night school, and is trying to parent three children under the age of five, life is stressful! When we feel stressed, our modern brains react just as the brains of our cave-dwelling ancestors did, releasing chemicals into the bloodstream to help us confront the stress (fight) or run away (flight). Over time, these same chemicals cause wear and tear on the body.

Defining Stress

Physician Hans Selye is responsible for much of our current understanding of stress. Just over fifty years ago he defined stress as the way the body responds to the demands placed on it, whether those demands are positive or negative. In Selye's terms, positive stress is *eustress* and negative stress is *distress* (1976).

Distress is what we usually think of when we think of stress—being yelled at by a boss, losing your job, financial difficulties, relationship issues, and so on. Distress is more detrimental than eustress, causing most of the wear and tear on our bodies. Eustress is stress that is considered helpful, either because it motivates us or because it makes us feel fulfilled. Examples include getting married, having a baby, winning the lottery, preparing for a physical challenge (e.g., a charity walk, a triathlon, or a championship game), and riding a roller coaster.

Stress can either be acute and short-lived or chronic. The top ten causes of stress include examples of both eustress and distress (Holmes and Rahe 1967):

1. Death of spouse

2. Divorce

3. Marital separation from mate

4. Detention in jail or other institution

5. Death of a close family member

6. Major personal injury or illness

7. Marriage

8. Being fired from your job

9. Marital reconciliation with mate

10. Retirement from work

Selye coined the term *stressor* to indicate anything that produces a stress response or disrupts the body's homeostasis or balance. Selye also described what he called the *general adaptation syndrome* (GAS)—the changing response of the body to stress over time, from onset to the continuous presence of stress to a chronic condition (1976).

The General Adaptation Syndrome: Fight vs. Flight

The GAS describes how the nervous system and the endocrine (hormonal) system respond to stressors, whether they are short-lived or persist and become chronic. All of these responses begin in the brain and then spread to the rest of the body. The three stages of the GAS are alarm (acute stress—occurs within minutes or hours of a stressful event), resistance (occurs within days or weeks), and exhaustion (occurs within weeks or months of the original stressful event).

ALARM

The body reacts immediately to an acute stressor by producing adrenaline and noradrenaline, which help the body prepare for either a fight or flight. The stress chemicals of this stage accelerate the heart rate, increase breathing, sharpen vision, and redirect blood flow to the muscles needed to fight or run away. Other symptoms of acute stress include tightness in the chest, sweaty palms, nausea, and dizziness.

RESISTANCE

When a stressful situation continues beyond an initial event, the body adapts to the ongoing stressor. However, in the process, the body's ability to resist new stressors decreases. For example, if you have BED/CO and are dieting or eating poorly—both of which stress the body—you may become ill if other stressors arise, overwhelming your body's coping mechanism. Symptoms of this stage include fatigue, irritability, depression, headaches, mood swings, food cravings, desires for drugs or alcohol, panic attacks, and changes in appetite.

EXHAUSTION

If a stressor becomes chronic, the body's reserves will be depleted, leading to wear and tear on the body. When you're under stress, your adrenal glands release large amounts of *cortisol*, a steroid hormone, to help keep your body going. Over time, high levels of cortisol can lead to what are sometimes called "diseases of adaptation," including heart attacks, autoimmune diseases (such as lupus, thyroid disease, and rheumatoid arthritis), cancer, post-traumatic stress disorder, and chronic depression.

As the GAS outlines, stress is actually a continuum, ranging from acute to chronic. Acute stress—the most common form of stress—is a short-lived response to an immediate perceived threat. Examples of acute eustress include taking a final exam, giving birth to a baby, or proposing to someone. Examples of acute distress include being in an automobile accident or getting a traffic ticket. Chronic eustress can result from raising children or working a demanding but satisfying job. Chronic distress can arise from a chronic illness—including eating disorders—either in yourself or in a loved one, or being in a job or marriage that is dissatisfying.

Acute and Chronic Stressors and Symptoms You've Experienced

We each have our own unique reactions to stress. Use the following chart to list acute and chronic stressors that you've experienced and any physical or emotional symptoms you experienced with them.

	Stressful Situation	Physical or Emotional Symptoms
Acute Stressors	Example: *I had a car accident.*	*Heart racing, sweaty, dry mouth.*

Chronic Stressors	Example: *My son's depression.*	*Tired all the time, more migraines, high blood pressure.*

HOW STRESS, DEPRESSION, TRAUMA, AND ADDICTIONS ARE LINKED IN THOSE WITH BED/CO

If you have BED or CO, you may have a hyperactive, or easily triggered, stress response. In other words, your body may be on red alert pretty much all of the time. This hyperactivity may have been caused by an experience of major stress in early childhood, trauma, abuse, or neglect. Being on red alert all the time makes you overreact to minor situations (NIH Backgrounder 2002) and can increase your likelihood of developing chronic diseases associated with stress. In those with BED, this hyperactive stress response is associated with increased appetite and bingeing (Gluck, Geliebter, and Lorence 2004). This hyperactivity is also linked to depression, addiction, and a history of trauma in people with BED/CO.

Let's explore this relationship further. (Therapies used to treat the conditions discussed are described in the next chapter.)

Trauma and Post-Traumatic Stress Disorder (PTSD)

Trauma is one of many experiences that can activate the stress response. Approximately 83 percent of people with BED report some form of childhood trauma, abuse, or neglect (Grilo et al. 2001; Allison et al., 2007). People who've been physically abused in childhood are twice as likely to develop an eating disorder than those with no history of abuse. This risk becomes even higher when there has been both physical and sexual abuse, rising to a threefold risk of developing an eating disorder (Rayworth, Wise, and Harlow 2004).

When trauma is severe, it can cause *post-traumatic stress disorder* (PTSD). PTSD can develop after an experience in which you—or someone else—was threatened with grave physical harm. You may have felt intense fear, helplessness, or horror, as well as increased arousal (red alert). Individuals with PTSD typically have recurrent memories of the traumatic experience; these may include nightmares or flashbacks that may be triggered by someone or something reminiscent of the event. As a result, people with PTSD may try to avoid anything that reminds them of the traumatic experience, and may develop depression, feelings of hopelessness, and numbness (an inability to feel their emotions).

Hyperarousal is the result of excessive, repetitive release of norepinephrine and epinephrine in response to situations or people that trigger trauma memories (Vanitallie 2002). Symptoms of increased arousal include insomnia, difficulty concentrating, increased anger, and being easily startled or overly vigilant. Individuals with a history of trauma may also experience depression, which may be partly due to the effect of the stress hormones on the limbic system, the part of the brain that helps us feel pleasure (Claes 2004).

PTSD can both contribute to the development of BED/CO and affect its symptoms. Individuals with a history of PTSD are more likely to engage in dysfunctional eating patterns, which can then worsen under stressful situations (Smyth et al. 2008). In both male and female military veterans, PTSD was found to increase the risk of being overweight or obese (Vieweg 2007; Dobie 2004). Having PTSD can also exacerbate eating disorders. For example, in one study, researchers found that obese binge eaters with a history of sexual and physical abuse became anorexic after undergoing a medical procedure they considered traumatic (Tobin, Molteni, and Elin 1995). If you have PTSD or a history of trauma, you may self-medicate feelings of anxiety or fear by bingeing or overeating; or you may engage in other unhealthy behaviors such as compulsive sexual behavior or the abuse of drugs, alcohol, or cigarettes (Zakarian et al. 2000).

Stress and Depression

Stress can cause depression. Both stress and depression can affect levels of the neurotransmitter serotonin and of stress hormones such as cortisol. Depression caused by chronic stress involves overproduction of cortisol; symptoms can include anxiety, aggressiveness, and difficulty tolerating traumatic life events. For people under chronic stress, depression should be treated not just with medication, but also with a strong focus on stress reduction (van Praag 2005).

Stress can also trigger depression, particularly in people with a family history of depression (Firk and Marksu 2007), as it decreases the level of serotonin in the brain—which in turn makes it more difficult to cope with stressors. Early life experiences and traumas can lead to a hyperactive stress response system and higher than normal production of cortisol. Elevated cortisol levels may contribute, either directly or indirectly, to the development of depression (van Praag 2005). Fortunately, stress-related depression can be successfully treated with integrative medicine; we'll discuss this in detail in the next chapter.

Stress and Addiction

The same chemicals involved in stress reactions and mood disorders are also involved in food cravings and drug and alcohol addictions. Many individuals with BED/CO are also addicted to drugs and/or alcohol. This isn't surprising. Different types of cravings may be accompanied by very similar obsessive thoughts and feelings of loss of control (O'Brien et al. 1998). The area of the brain that drugs or alcohol activate in addicts is also activated in women with eating disorders in response to food stimuli, which may explain some of the compulsive aspects of eating disorders (Uher et al. 2004). When naloxone—a medication used to block the pleasurable effects of narcotics on the brain—was given to women who were binge eaters, there was a significant reduction in preference for typical comfort foods (sweet, high-fat foods), much more than when given to people without a history of bingeing (Drenowski et al. 1995).

Stress and Food Cravings

You may have noticed for yourself that you eat more of certain foods—or just more food—when stressed. A survey done by the American Institute for Cancer Research found that in the months immediately after the terrorist attacks of 9/11 people ate more comfort foods (2001). About 20 percent of those surveyed reported eating more mashed potatoes with gravy, friend chicken, and macaroni and cheese than previously. There was also an increase in cravings for foods such as cookies and ice cream. Specific types of food cravings can be cultural. For example, researchers found that women in Japan are more likely to crave rice and sushi than sweet, high-fat foods (Komatsu 2008).

Many people crave rich foods when under stress. Eating such foods may actually be a coping mechanism our bodies use to deal with stressful times. High-fat, sweet comfort foods trigger the release of brain chemicals that make us feel better, including serotonin, also affected by antidepressant medications. In animal models, comfort foods have been found to help shut off the fight versus flight mechanism, calming our bodies down after a red alert (Dallman et al. 2003).

Other research has found that when rats are exposed to both stress and dieting, they become binge eaters, although neither stress nor dieting by itself is enough to cause them to binge. In addition, stimulation of the brain's reward system can cause rats to binge even when well-fed. This finding suggests that bingeing may be driven by an urge to attain a reward (i.e., the release of feel-good brain chemicals), rather than hunger or metabolic need; this may also explain why eating even a small amount of a trigger food can lead to a binge. The researchers who conducted this study suggest that rats who are dieting or are under stress may be in a state of pleasure deprivation and therefore more vulnerable to cravings (Boggiano et al. 2007).

Stress can affect our choice of food, shifting our choices from lower-fat to higher-fat items. Under stress, food consumption is increased in women more than men. Of those who overeat under stress, 71 percent are dieters; the foods eaten under stress tend to be the foods they avoid when dieting (high-calorie, high-fat snack foods); they report that eating these foods makes them feel better when under stress (Zellner 2006).

Food Cravings

On the left side of the following table, list any foods that you crave under stress. On the right side, describe what need these foods fulfill when you're under stress. If you're not sure, start by describing a food's texture, flavor, and other qualities. How does the food make you feel? What purpose does it serve in your life?

Food You Crave Under Stress	What the Food Means to You
Example: *Strawberry shortcake.*	*Strawberry shortcake reminds me of being in my grandmother's kitchen, where I always felt safe.*

Now that you have a sense of the emotional purposes these foods may serve, next time you have a craving see if you can feed your emotional need in a different way. In the following table, list first the emotional needs you've identified through working with the previous table—the need for safety, nurturing, love, attention, and so on—and then other ways of meeting that need.

Emotional Need	Other Ways to Meet This Need
Example: *The need to feel nurtured.*	*I could take a hot bubble bath with aromatherapy bath salts and candles.* *I could get a massage.*

Can Stress Make You Gain Weight?

Stress itself can promote weight gain through a number of complex factors:

* Poor quality of sleep: Poor or unrefreshing sleep due to stress can contribute to weight gain. When you don't sleep well, the stress hormone cortisol is released at a higher level, making you feel hungrier. As well, poor sleep can inhibit the release of a growth hormone, making it harder to lose fat and grow calorie-burning muscle tissue.

* Depression: Stress can cause depression, which can increase appetite and decrease activity levels in some individuals.

* Changes in diet: We eat different foods—more high-fat, sweet foods—when under stress; these foods typically have a greater number of calories, increasing the likelihood of weight gain.

Recognizing that stress can exacerbate bingeing and overeating can allow you to better prepare for stressful times and be more conscious of your eating choices when under stress.

BRINGING IT ALL TOGETHER

As we've seen, stress can have a substantial negative impact on many different aspects of your life. However, becoming more aware of stress can improve both your health and your well-being.

Identify Your Level of Stress

For one week, use the following table to rate your level of stress, with 0 equal to no stress at all (i.e., you've been sent to a planet where there isn't even the concept of stress and all of your desires are immediately taken care of), and 10 equal to off the charts stress. Do the same for your food cravings, with 0 equal to no food cravings at all that day, and 10 equal to a day spent completely and painfully obsessed with the Oreo cookies in your pantry at home.

Next, describe your emotional state or mood. Use whatever words are appropriate—depressed, down, anxious, sad, happy, fearful, guilty, shameful, angry, and so on. Finally, list any specific foods you craved.

	Level of Stress (0–10)	Food Craving (0–10)	Mood	Specific Foods Craved
Monday				
Tuesday				
Wednesday				
Thursday				
Friday				
Saturday				
Sunday				

Rating your stress level and food cravings for a week or longer can help you identify patterns specific to your individual food, mood, and stress issues. For example, you may discover that Fridays are always high in work stress, that you can't wait to go out with friends once the workday has ended—and that when you do, you typically drink and eat more than you'd like. Or perhaps you go home after your tough workday and binge on ice cream in front of the television. We'll work with such patterns in the next exercise.

Your Stress-Eating Patterns

Look at your notes from the week you tracked. What patterns can you identify? Next to each pattern, list one small thing you can do to change it—anything that will help you stop using food to deal with stress or fill emotional needs. (We'll discuss tools to help you cope with stress in greater detail in the next chapter.)

Stress-Eating Pattern	A Healthy Way to Change This Pattern
Example: *When I have a work deadline, my stress level goes up, and I always buy a dozen donuts to take to work with me. Although I share the donuts, I always end up eating most of them.*	*When I have a stressful deadline, I will buy only two donuts to take with me, and make a date to do something fun after work so I have something to look forward to.*

Good work! You are continuing to make changes that you can sustain. (Remember: it is by taking small, sustainable steps that you create long-term, enduring change.) As you can see, learning how to manage stress is an important part of your recovery process. Lowering your reaction to stressful events can actually affect both your weight and your eating patterns.

WHAT DOES STRESS MEAN TO YOU?

We've explored at length what experts know about stress and how it affects your health and well-being. Now it's time to make this all a bit more personal. Some of the things that really stress you out personally may not seem to bother other people—and some things that really bother others may not ruffle your feathers even the slightest bit. Everyday stressors in your life may add up and contribute to depression, hopelessness, and feeling overwhelmed—and to disordered eating. On the other hand, you may be less reactive to stress if you are well-rested and feel self-confident because other areas of your life are going well. Use the following exercise to explore how you personally experience stress.

How Do You Experience Stress?

There are many different ways of coping with stress. Your answers to the following questions will help you determine how you personally tend to react to stress:

1.	Do you often feel tension in your neck or shoulders?	YES	NO
2.	Do you experience pain in your jaw in the morning, or notice that you clench your jaw during the day?	YES	NO
3.	Do you often eat when not hungry?	YES	NO
4.	Do you often feel impatient (e.g., tapping your foot or pacing)?	YES	NO
5.	Do you have trouble falling asleep because your mind is racing?	YES	NO
6.	Do you have trouble controlling your anger?	YES	NO
7.	Do you have heart palpitations, frequent urination, or lower back pain?	YES	NO
8.	Do you tend to cry more easily than you used to?	YES	NO
9.	Do you often feel overwhelmed?	YES	NO
10.	Do you sometimes feel like life "just isn't worth it"?	YES	NO
11.	Do you often feel as if your problems are much worse than other people's?	YES	NO
12.	Have you recently started smoking again after quitting?	YES	NO
13.	Do you find yourself drinking more than usual or wanting to drink more often?	YES	NO
14.	Have you been more promiscuous lately?	YES	NO
15.	Have you been isolating yourself more than usual?	YES	NO
16.	Do you tend to crave sweets?	YES	NO

Somaticization: If you answered yes to questions 1, 2, 3, 7, and 16 in the preceding exercise, you may *somaticize* your stress. In other words, you may feel most of your stress in your body, perhaps even becoming physically ill when under stress. For you, it's important to pay close attention to physical cues that signal that your stress level is higher than normal. Also, take extra care of your body when under stress—sleep well, eat nourishing food, and avoid becoming physically exhausted.

Nervous system activation: If you answered yes to questions 4, 5, 6, and 14, you may tend to experience stress as nervous system activation—that is, you become jittery or anxious and have trouble sitting still or sleeping. In essence, stress gets you very wound up; as a result, you may make rash or impulsive decisions. If this describes you, establish escape valves for use when stress levels become high. For example, to release emotion you might call a close friend or go to a movie where you can have a good cry; when you anticipate a stressful period, you might schedule regular massages. Don't allow stress levels to become so high that you explode emotionally.

Moodiness: If you answered yes to questions 8, 9, 10, 11, 12, 13, and 15, you may express your stress through your moods. You may find yourself depressed, tearful, or feeling overwhelmed when stress levels get high. If so, it's important for you to guard against your emotions taking control of you. If stress causes you to have more pessimistic or negative thoughts, get help with your mood quickly, before depression sets in. You may want to consult a therapist at the first sign of a lowering of your mood. Several alternative therapies, such as energy medicine, supplements, and acupuncture can also help. We'll discuss these in the following chapter.

You may have answered yes to questions in more than one category. That's okay: you don't have to fit into just one category. Perhaps with minor stressors you have one type of response, while with major stressors you have another. What's important is to be aware of how stress affects you so you can be proactive in addressing stress and better cope with stressful times.

SUMMARY

Stress, mood, trauma, and eating patterns share important connections. It's critical to both recognize the signs and symptoms of stress and understand the impact stress can have on your life—this will improve your ability to cope with stress in healthy rather than unhealthy ways. The next step is enhancing your skills. In the following chapter, we'll add more ways to cope with stress to your toolbox, including both conventional methods and complementary and alternative techniques.

CHAPTER 11

Tools to Manage Stress

Various strategies can help you reduce unhealthy reactions to stress—and thus lower the health risks associated with stress. These strategies include both basic stress management techniques that help reduce your vulnerability to stress as well as therapies from complementary and alternative medicine (CAM). CAM therapies are particularly helpful in dealing with stress because many work directly on the stress reaction, lowering stress hormone levels and inducing deep states of relaxation that counteract the fight versus flight response. In addition, certain mind-body practices can help you avoid some stressors and cope better with those you cannot. At the end of this chapter, after we've discussed these different strategies in detail, you'll have a chance to put together your own personal stress management plan.

BASIC STRESS MANAGEMENT STRATEGIES

When we're tired or ill, we don't handle stress as well as when we're at the peak of health. Indeed, if you're already under high stress—for whatever reason—when yet another stressor comes your way, you're likely to have more trouble dealing with it than if you weren't stressed at all. We can see this in Sara's story:

Sara, a twenty-seven-year-old executive assistant, is often tired and disheartened at work because she doesn't feel appreciated by her boss or allowed to express her creativity. She tends to deal with these feelings by overeating and snacking, then going on a diet, then returning to overeating. She is the single mother of Evan, a two-year-old little boy who takes up most of her off-time. Recently, Sara fell and fractured her left wrist and was told she would need a cast for six weeks. The following day, Evan developed a fever at daycare and Sara had to leave work to pick him up. Sara's boss was upset about the days Sara was going to have to be absent to care for Evan, which added further to Sara's stress. When, the next day, Sara's mother called and asked if Sara could give her a ride to a doctor's appointment—something Sara had happily done in the past—something inside Sara snapped. She yelled, "Why do I have to do everything for you? Don't you know you're not the only one with problems?" and slammed down the phone, bursting into tears.

Does Sara's story sound familiar? Often life's stresses come at us without warning, sometimes without end. Therefore, it is important to be as prepared as you can be to meet whatever challenges come your way. One crucial element to accomplishing this is to be as physically strong and resilient as possible. The three must-haves for staying strong and healthy—sleep, nutrition, and exercise—are all practices that are under your control. Let's explore each of these in greater detail.

Getting a Good Night's Sleep

You may not consider sleep a top priority. Like many Americans, you may shave time from your sleep to finish a project at work, catch up on your cleaning, or care for your children, partner, or friends. Although sleep needs are different for different individuals, most sleep experts recommend that adults get between seven and eight hours of sleep a night (WebMD 2008).

It is also important that your sleep be of good quality. For many of us, it is not. If you are a new parent, your sleep is likely to be frequently interrupted; as a result you may wake up in the morning feeling as if you haven't slept enough or at all. Or your sleep may be of poor quality for other reasons. For example, if you suffer from gastroesophageal reflux disease (GERD or acid reflux disease), periodic limb movements in sleep (PLMS) (formerly known as restless legs syndrome), or sleep apnea, your sleep may be interrupted during the night. Fortunately, all of these conditions can be treated, enabling you to get a good night's sleep.

It is particularly critical to focus on getting enough high-quality sleep if you have BED/CO and are overweight or obese. Obese people have a higher incidence of insomnia, excessive daytime sleepiness, and other general sleep problems. Obese individuals also report a higher incidence of emotional stress in their lives than non-obese individuals; this is then exacerbated by poor sleep (Vgontzas et al. 2008). The relationship between sleep, stress, and weight cannot be overemphasized.

You may think you're doing fine with just four or five hours of sleep a night. But remember: not getting enough sleep increases your risk of obesity. Also, people who sleep less than six hours per night for more than a week display the same cognitive deficits as those who haven't slept at all for two days straight. These cognitive deficits include not being able to react effectively to stimuli (e.g., while driving); reduced problem-solving capabilities, and the inability to perform several tasks at the same time. Most people who are experiencing cognitive deficits do not even realize they are impaired. Research suggests that to avoid these deficits, the average person needs 8.16 hours of sleep per night (Van Dongen et al. 2003).

Improve Your Sleep Habits

Review the following list of habits that promote good sleep. Mark those you presently possess. For habits you want to adopt or improve, describe what actions you will take.

Sleep Habit	Yes/No	Changes You Want to Make
You have a ritual for sleep; go to bed and get up at the same time.		
You don't exercise rigorously or do taxing mental work right before bedtime.		
Your bedroom is quiet, peaceful, and dark.		
You don't drink alcohol in order to fall asleep.		
You don't fall asleep with the TV on or watch TV right before bed.		
You don't use the bedroom for any activities other than sleep and sex.		
You don't go to bed hungry or overfull.		
If you take a daytime nap, it is for less than a hour.		

If you tend to wake up at night worrying, keep a notepad beside your bed; write down your worries in it before you go to sleep and whenever you wake up at night. If you don't dream at night, you may not be getting enough sleep. If sleep problems persist, discuss them with your health care provider.

NATURAL SLEEP AIDS

Several over-the-counter herbal products can help you sleep. (If you are taking any prescription medications, please speak with your medical provider before taking herbs or other over-the-counter sleep aids.) If you are unsure of which brand to try, ask your pharmacist or health care provider for advice. No sleep aid should be taken every night; taken on a short-term basis, however, sleep aids can help restore a healthy sleep pattern.

Valerian: This herb has been used for decades. Before the onset of current prescription sleep medicines, valerian was the most common sleep medicine prescribed by doctors. Many studies have supported its efficacy.

5-Hydroxytryptophan (5-HTP): 5-HTP is converted to serotonin (a brain chemical increased by many antidepressant medications) in the brain. It helps deepen sleep and restore dreams and has been used to treat insomnia, as well as depression, anxiety, obesity, and fibromyalgia.

Melatonin: Although melatonin is best known for restoring sleep after jet lag or other circadian rhythm disturbances—for example, late-night work shifts—it can also help you fall asleep more quickly and may improve quality of sleep (Simpson and Curran 2008).

Natural Sleep Aids: Dosages, Side Effects, and Cautions

Herb	Dose	Side Effects	Cautions
Valerian	900 milligrams thirty minutes before bedtime.	May cause headaches, upset stomach, dizziness, and low body temperature.	Should not be used during pregnancy or while breastfeeding. If you are on a prescription antidepressant, consult your doctor before taking, as it may interact with some antidepressant medications. Do not take with medications that are sedating or while driving.
5-HTP	Starting dose is 50 milligrams up to 200 milligrams at bedtime.	May cause heartburn, stomachaches, nausea, and diarrhea.	Persons with bipolar disorder should not take 5-HTP except under supervision of their health care professional, as it may trigger mania. If you are on a prescription antidepressant, consult your doctor before taking, as it may interact with some antidepressant medications.
Melatonin	0.3–5.0 milligrams.	Daytime drowsiness, headache, dizziness.	May interact with blood thinning medications, other sedatives, diabetic medications and alcohol. Do not take if you are undergoing cancer therapy or on immunosuppressive drugs.

Eating Patterns, Nutrition, and Stress

You've already learned most of what you need to know about nutrition in preceding chapters. Let's focus now on how eating patterns—as well as what you do or don't eat—can affect your ability to cope with stress.

EATING PATTERNS THAT WORSEN STRESS

The following are some common eating patterns that you may fall into when under stress:

Starting a new diet. While it may seem like a good idea to start a new diet when you're going through a stressful time, any type of diet is stressful. This is true whether you're resolving to fast during the day, eat only one meal a day, or throw out all the junk food and start a whole new healthy eating plan. When you're under stress, the best approach is to make tiny changes. For example, decrease the number of sodas you drink a day from ten to eight. Or better yet, just resolve to eat an extra fruit or vegetable a day. Wait to embark on larger changes until you are less stressed emotionally so as to avoid stressing yourself physically.

Eating more junk food than usual. It's not uncommon to feel hungrier under stress. The extra cortisol in your bloodstream from the stress reaction can increase food cravings, especially cravings for sweets and high-fat foods. Eating sweets can increase serotonin in our brains, which makes us feel good—but so can taking a walk. Most importantly, if you do yield to your craving, eat mindfully, with your attention focused on how the food tastes and on how it feels in your mouth and your body. Mindless eating tends to lead to overeating or bingeing; by staying focused on what you're eating, you're less likely to let emotions or stress control how much and what you eat.

Losing your appetite, only to have it come back later with a vengeance. Although you may not feel hungry when dealing with a big stressor like the breakup of a relationship, don't stop eating, as this can increase your bingeing later on. Instead, eat small meals or snacks throughout the day to avoid rebound hunger.

Eating because your appetite is out of control. If you feel like overeating, first check your level of hunger. Ask yourself what you're really hungry for (emotionally). What (emotions) are you trying to stuff down with your food? See if you can satisfy the craving or emotional need in another way. If you're not sure what you're really hungry for, try using one of the distraction techniques discussed in chapter 5; this can help you identify if your hunger is physical or emotional. For example, drink a glass of water, call a friend, or take a walk. Stay mindful of what your body needs as opposed to what you need emotionally and respond accordingly.

Eating because you feel tired. When you're stressed to the max, you may feel tired and have low energy. Don't mistake this for true physical hunger. Eating won't raise your energy in this instance; in fact, eating large amounts of food can actually further stress your body because it diverts scarce energy resources to digestion. Test whether or not you're physically hungry by eating a small snack and paying attention to your body's cues. If you find that you're just tired, then take a nap or engage in some other restful activity.

Eating Patterns Under Stress

Mark the patterns you identify with when you are under stress: (You may identify with more than one.)

Starting a new diet when stressed out.

Increasing your consumption of junk foods.

Losing your appetite only to later have it go out of control.

Overeating because your appetite has gone up dramatically.

Eating more because you feel tired.

Other: _____

Other: _____

Other: _____

List three telltale signs that will help you identify the patterns you've listed above: (Example: *I know I'm stress-eating when I stop at a fast food restaurant on the way home and eat in my car. Or: I know I'm going to binge when I get home from work when I haven't eaten all day.*)

1. _____

2. _____

3. _____

List actions you can take when these signs indicate that you are stress-eating: (Example: *If I find myself craving fast food, I'll make dinner plans with a friend and talk about my stressful day. Or: When I realize I've skipped breakfast, I'll make sure to eat a healthy lunch and a mid-morning protein snack to avoid bingeing later in the evening.*)

_____

_____

_____

_____

_____

Nutrition Guidelines for Stress Reduction

Certain foods help your body deal with stress while others make coping with stress all the more difficult. Foods to avoid when under stress include sugar, caffeine, alcohol, and high-fat items. Foods that can help support your body when under stress include healthy fats (such as those found in avocados, olive oil, and canola oil); immune system–boosting fish (salmon, mackerel, and tuna); and nuts, which are chock full of B vitamins. Research has found that consumption of foods rich in calcium and vitamin D—such as low-fat milk—may help reduce symptoms of premenstrual tension (Bertone-Johnson et al. 2005); vitamin D also supports healthy immune function under stress.

DIETARY SUPPLEMENTS FOR STRESS

Over time, stress depletes the body's levels of magnesium, B vitamins, and vitamins A and C. Eating foods rich in these nutrients supports your body during stress. Even small deficits of these nutrients can affect your nervous system—and therefore your ability to cope with stress. For example, magnesium deficiency can cause stress-related depression, sensitivity to noise, and irritability (Somer 1999). During times of stress—either acute or chronic—consider supplementing your diet with vitamins and minerals that will offer your body support. (*Note:* Magnesium should be taken with calcium to avoid an imbalance in either; I usually recommend taking 450 milligrams of magnesium in tandem with 1000 milligrams of calcium for those under fifty or 1200 milligrams for those over fifty.) If you have a medical condition or are on medication, consult your health care provider before taking supplements.

In addition to the nutrients already mentioned, other nutrients to seek out include chromium, copper, and omega-3 fatty acids. Chromium helps regulate blood sugar; swings in blood sugar can exacerbate food cravings and bingeing. Food sources of chromium include romaine lettuce, raw onions, and tomatoes; to a lesser degree, chromium is also found in whole grains, bran cereals, potatoes, oysters, and liver.

Copper has many useful functions: it is involved in the production of blood cells, protects against free-radical damage, promotes good sleep, and is anti-inflammatory. Food sources include sesame seeds, sunflower seeds, raw cashews, cooked barley, cooked tempeh, garbanzo beans, navy beans, cooked soybeans, raw crimini mushrooms, and calf's liver.

Omega-3 fatty acids were discussed in detail in chapter 3. They can help stabilize mood, lower blood pressure, and reduce levels of stress hormones (Mills et al. 1989). Food sources include fish (salmon, tuna, halibut), fish oils, seeds, seed oils, walnuts, nut oils, soybeans, and marine life such as algae and krill.

HERBS FOR STRESS: THE ADAPTOGENS

Adaptogens are herbs that help your body adapt to stress by restoring homeostasis (balance) and supporting the adrenal glands as they work overtime to produce stress hormones in response to the stress reaction.

Because adaptogens are herbs, their doses are based on extracts containing a standard percentage of the active ingredient. When selecting an herbal product, check its percentage of the active ingredient (this will be listed on the bottle or packing material). Two adaptogens to consider if you find yourself in a stressful period are ginseng and Rhodiola rosea.

Ginseng. In addition to helping the body deal with stress, ginseng also supports the immune system and is thought to promote longevity. *Panax ginseng*, native to Asia, is used in Chinese medicine to treat anxiety, insomnia, restlessness, and stomach disturbances associated with mental and nervous exhaustion. American ginseng (*Panax quinquefolius*), native to North America, is very similar to *Panax ginseng*. Studies have found that ginseng enhances mental performance (Sorensen and Sonne 1996) and can help lower blood sugar in type 2 (non-insulin dependent) diabetics (Sotaniemi 1995). Interestingly, ginseng increases blood sugar in those with low levels; thus, for individuals with BED/CO who have diabetes or metabolic syndrome, ginseng may help stabilize blood sugar levels, and thereby decrease cravings. Ginseng is used to treat prolonged stress, exhaustion, chronic fatigue syndrome, and mild depression as well as to aid recovery from illness and surgery. The usual dose of the dried root is 0.5 to 3.0 milligrams, containing at least 1.5 percent ginsenosides. Tinctures (liquid preparations) are standardized to 4 percent ginsenosides, with a usual starting dose of 200–400 milligrams once or twice daily; doses up to 4 grams per day can be used safely. Toxicity is seen only when excessive amounts are taken (more than 4 grams/day). Ginseng use should be limited to three months at a time. If you are diabetic, use with caution because ginseng may lower blood glucose. If you have been diagnosed with breast cancer, take ginseng only under the supervision of a health care practitioner as there is a theoretical possibility it can stimulate estrogen-like activity in women. Do not take with coffee or tea. Ginseng may be stimulating in higher doses and can cause insomnia.

Rhodiola rosea. Also known as roseroot or golden root, Rhodiola rosea has been taken for centuries in Russia, including by Russian cosmonauts. It is used to increase physical endurance and to treat fatigue, depression, and anxiety. Rhodiola both promotes the release of brain chemicals that affect our mood and has antioxidant properties that help our bodies deal with the inflammation caused by stress. Start with 50 milligrams (standardized to 3 percent rosavins) and increase slowly, up to 200 milligrams per day. If you suffer from anxiety you may experience an increase in anxiety symptoms; if you decrease the dose this will improve. If you have been diagnosed with bipolar depression, take Rhodiola only under a health care practitioner's supervision in order to avoid precipitating mania.

Exercise for Stress Reduction

Exercise can be a useful adjunct to other methods of handling stress. Exercise increases the production of endorphins in the brain, which helps elevate mood and improve quality of life (physical, emotional, and social well-being). The World Health Organization considers exercise to promote long-term health by improving workplace productivity and reducing risks for the medical conditions associated with prolonged stress, such as high blood pressure, heart disease, obesity, and diabetes (Briazgounov 1988). Because exercise boosts the immune system, people who exercise regularly are less likely to become sick after stressful events than those who don't (Fleshner 2005). Exercise can counteract the desire to binge or overeat that often accompanies periods of high stress by helping to regulate blood sugar levels (Somer 1999). Although the mechanism isn't clearly understood yet, researchers now know that exercise can also prevent the development of stress-related depression and anxiety (Greenwood and Fleshner 2008). In individuals diagnosed with post-traumatic stress disorder, aerobic exercise reduces symptoms associated with PTSD and trauma (Diaz and Motta 2008).

Studies have found that if you are overweight or obese but physically fit, your risk of death is lower than that of normal-weight persons who are not fit (Barlow et al. 1995; Blair and Brodney 1999). The Centers for Disease Control recommend thirty minutes of moderate-intensity exercise almost every day for better health (2002).

Most of these benefits can be achieved through aerobic exercise and increasing your level of physical activity (for example, by taking the stairs instead of the elevator). However, bear in mind that exercise can also be a stressor. When you force yourself to exercise—or push yourself to the point of exhaustion—you add to the stress your body has to deal with rather than reduce it.

YOGA AND TAI CHI

Yoga is an element of Ayurvedic medicine, a traditional system of healing from India. Ayurveda uses yoga, meditation, herbs, and dietary therapies to treat and prevent illness. Tai chi, a form of martial arts, is the most popular form of qigong, which originated in traditional Chinese medicine (TCM) and has been practiced by millions of people in Asia for health maintenance and disease prevention.

The benefits of both yoga and tai chi lie in their ability to reunite mind and body. Both combine breathwork and meditation (to calm the mind) with a series of movements that encourage strength and flexibility (to calm the body). The control of breathing found in both yoga and tai chi promotes relaxation and stress reduction (Ross 2007).

If you're not familiar with either yoga or tai chi you may feel intimidated by the strangeness of these forms of exercise. If you are overweight, you may worry that you won't be able to perform the different movements. If either of these is the case, consider starting with a few private lessons with a skilled teacher. Yoga and tai chi classes are now offered at most fitness clubs, wellness centers, and YMCA and YWCA clubs. If your goal is stress reduction, ask if the class you're interested in is suitable for this purpose. Some classes are focused less on relaxation and more on vigorous exercise.

In the following exercise, list any physical activities that you currently do that help you deal with stress, as well as additional forms of exercise you want to try. Be adventurous! Find activities that you look forward to, even if it's just walking around a local park. Look for exercises and activities that you find relaxing.

Stress-Reducing Exercise

List any physical exercises you currently do that are stress reducing:

_____

_____

_____

_____

_____

Next, mark any activities you would like to try or learn more about:

Yoga

Tai chi

Swimming

Skating

Biking or joining a bike club (these exist for all skill levels)

Pilates

Weight training

Sailing

Martial arts

Nature walks or hikes

Dancing

Other:

_____

_____

_____

Physical activity and exercise can help you relax and be more mindful in your daily life. Find things you enjoy doing and that make you feel good—you're more likely to continue doing them.

HEALING THERAPIES FOR STRESS MANAGEMENT

The category of complementary and alternative medicine (CAM) includes numerous therapies. Many have been proved through scientific research; many are supported by thousands of years of experiential evidence. Let's focus now on those therapies that have the greatest impact on stress reactions. (See the resources section at the back of the book for websites that will help you learn more about the different therapies and find qualified practitioners in your area. Other good sources for referrals are family and friends and training centers for these techniques.) I have found all of the CAM therapies that follow helpful in treating individuals with BED/CO.

In many traditional systems of healing, disease—or "dis-ease"—is viewed as the result of imbalances in your body, mind, and spirit. Stress is one of the many causes of such imbalances. Various CAM therapies can help you rebalance yourself—calm your racing mind or heart, decrease your exhaustion, and refocus your concentration. By rebalancing yourself—physically, spiritually, and mentally—you can reduce the harmful effects of stress and increase your body's ability to heal from whatever stressors have caused the imbalances.

Massage Therapy

Massage therapy (covered in more depth in chapter 9) promotes restorative sleep and calms the symptoms of the stress response, reducing levels of stress hormones and increasing levels of dopamine and serotonin (Field et al. 2005).

Acupuncture

Acupuncture (also discussed in chapter 9) has been approved by the World Health Organization as a treatment for stress (Bannerman 1979). Research has found that acupuncture decreases the elevation in blood pressure that usually accompanies stress (Middlekauff, Yu, and Hui 2001).

Chiropractic

Chiropractic therapies have been around for two hundred years. Chiropractic is based on the fact the all of the major nerves that send impulses to the different parts of the body—including the brain—come through the spinal column. The underlying philosophy of chiropractic is that if your spinal column is out of alignment, the nervous system will not function at its highest capacity. (Manipulation of the spinal column has been a component of many traditional healing systems, dating back to ancient Greece.) As a result of stress or injury, you may experience muscle spasms in your neck, shoulders, and lower back. Chiropractic care can help reduce or eliminate the muscle spasms and tension often associated with stress.

Energy Medicine

Energy medicine is based on the idea that living beings are infused with vital energy. This energy or biofield is called by different names in different cultures: qi (chi) in China, ki in Japan, and prana in India. Although this vital energy is difficult to measure, we know it exists if only by seeing its absence in organisms that are no longer alive. Energy healers believe that a disturbance in the biofield causes of illness—and that by correcting this imbalance, health can be restored.

Therapeutic touch, johrei, polarity therapy, zero balancing, and reiki are all forms of energy work that help the body and mind enter deep states of restorative relaxation. Researchers have studied therapeutic touch (TT) in a wide array of medical conditions, including osteoarthritis, headaches, anxiety, and wound healing. A review of ten studies of TT found a positive benefit in seven (Winstead-Fry and Kijek 1999). In regard to reiki, studies have found that it decreases heart rate and blood pressure (Mackay, Hansen, and McFarlane 2004) and reduces symptoms of psychological depression and self-perceived stress (Shore 2004).

MIND-BODY THERAPIES FOR STRESS MANAGEMENT

The scientific study of mind-body medicine is heavily influenced by the work of Herbert Benson, who in 1974 studied the relaxation response of individuals who practiced transcendental meditation. However, the understanding that the mind is important in healing goes back to Hippocrates, the father of modern medicine. Hippocrates argued that illness not only affects the body, it also has moral and spiritual aspects (National Center for Complementary and Alternative Medicine 2004). What all mind-body modalities have in common is the promotion of the relaxation response described by Benson (Lazar et al. 2000; Davidson et al. 2003). Therapies under this umbrella include meditation, breathwork, guided imagery, hypnosis, biofeedback, and relaxation training.

Benefits of mind-body therapies include improved immune function, lower cortisol levels, and improved attention abilities (Tang et al. 2007); improved quality of life, decreased stress symptoms, and beneficial changes in the effect of the stress response on the brain (Carlson et al. 2004); and improved mood and lower perceived stress (Lane, Seskevich, and Pieper 2007). For individuals with eating disorders, mind-body therapy can reduce symptoms of bingeing (Pop-Jordanova 2000; Esplen et al. 1998) and improve body image (Walsh 2008; Anbar and Savedoff 2005).

However, mind-body techniques are only useful when practiced. One way to do so is to include time for daily reflection in your life. As the old saying goes, stop and smell the roses—regularly. If you want to try out mind-body practices, breathwork offers an excellent way to slow the mind. Try this exercise:

Focus on Your Breath to Quiet the Mind

Find a quiet corner where you won't be interrupted, even if it's in the bathtub. Sit comfortably, placing your hands on your lower abdomen. If you're comfortable doing so, close your eyes. Now, take a deep breath, in through your nose and out through your mouth. As you breathe in, push your belly out against your hands. Feel it draw back in with your exhale. Next, for three breaths, breathe in to the count of four and out to the count of eight. This is harder than it sounds. Take your time—it gets easier with practice. Over time, increase the number of your breaths, from three to five, then eight, and so on. Stay seated when you've finished the process of conscious breathing. Allow your breath to gently return to its own rhythm. Stay aware of your breath until you feel relaxed.

You can do this exercise anywhere: at home, at work, while shopping. Breathwork is probably the most important daily practice you can engage in to reduce your stress level; it moves your attention out of your busy, stress-filled mind and into your body, giving you a moment of awareness and relaxation that refreshes both mind and body.

INTERPERSONAL PRACTICES FOR STRESS MANAGEMENT

Because stressors occur on a daily basis in all of our lives, it is important to have a plan in place that reduces stressors whenever possible and allows you to manage stress on a daily basis. Various interpersonal practices can help you counter stress through improving your relationships and social support system. Consider the following suggestions; add those that make sense for your life to your personal stress management plan at the end of this chapter.

Learn to Say No to Doing Too Much

Is your plate too full? Are you trying to please or take care of everyone else at your own expense? Over time, being overcommitted can cause a great deal of stress in your life. Saying no doesn't make you selfish; it makes you more able to spend quality time with the people who mean the most to you, including yourself. Use the following skills to help you reduce stress:

* Think very carefully before saying yes to long-term commitments (e.g., becoming chair of a fundraising event) as opposed to short-term commitments (e.g., baking cookies for a school function). Sleep on bigger commitments before making a decision.

* Have a list of priorities. Measure your commitments against your priorities. Knowing your priorities makes it easier to say no.

* Recognize when you're going overboard, then see what is actually required and do just that. Try doing less than what you think is expected; see what feedback you get.

* Practice saying no until you are comfortable doing so. Ask a person you trust to help you practice.

Develop a Strong Social Network

Social networks can include family and friends. Developing a social network takes time, and should be on your priority list. If you're too stressed out to connect with other people, reexamine your priorities right away. Maintaining a social network reduces stress; it doesn't cause it. That said, social networks are ideally developed when you're not under stress so that the relationships are in place when you need them. When developing a social network, choose people who are supportive and nonjudgmental. You may need to be the one who makes the first—or second or third—contact. As you recover from BED/ CO, it's also important to surround yourself with other recovery-minded individuals. One of the crucial elements of a good network is a respect for each other's privacy; this means no gossiping. And remember: always express your gratitude for those in your social network.

Now, let's bring together all you've learned in this chapter to create a cohesive plan for managing your personal stress.

Developing Your Personal Stress Management Plan

It's time to develop your personal approach to managing stress. This plan will be your template for successful stress management in the future; it can be modified and updated over time as you learn what works best for you.

List both whatever you are already doing to manage stress that works for you as well as habits you'd like to change or therapies you'd like to add to your stress management plan. Refer to earlier exercises to remind yourself of the areas you've identified as needing improvement.

Stress Management Tools	Action to Take
Example: *Basic stress management strategies: sleep, nutrition, and exercise (including yoga and tai chi)*	*I will sleep a minimum of seven hours a night; I will begin taking a multivitamin; I will take valerian for insomnia; I will walk fifteen minutes a day.*
Basic stress management strategies: sleep,* nutrition, and exercise (including yoga and tai chi)	
Nutritional supplements: magnesium (remember to balance with calcium), B vitamins, vitamin A, vitamin C, omega-3 fatty acids, chromium, copper	
Adaptogen herbs: Ginseng, Rhodiola rosea	
CAM therapies: massage, acupuncture, chiropractic, reiki, zero balancing, others	
Mind-body therapies: meditation, breathwork, guided imagery, hypnosis, biofeedback, and relaxation training	
Interpersonal stress strategies: learning to say no, building a support network	

*An excellent book on sleep is *Healing Night: The Science and Spirit of Sleeping, Dreaming, and Awakening* by Rubin Naiman (2006).

Next, write five goals you'd like to achieve in terms of stress management during the next six to twelve months: (Example: *I want to have two daily practices for reflection that I consistently do. I want to take at least two private yoga classes every week.*)

1. _____

2. _____

3. _____

4. _____

5. _____

SUMMARY

Stress is unavoidable—we're all prone to it. It is vital to recognize the signs of stress before it causes health problems for you, to be aware of your personal stressors, and to develop strategies for managing stress. For more information about using complementary and alternative therapies, supplements, and herbs for BED/CO, visit my website at www.carolynrossmd.com.

CHAPTER 12

Nourishing Your Spirit

In today's busy world, it's easy to forget the importance of nourishing our spirit. However, whether you call it spirit or soul or just the vital energy that distinguishes you as a living being from someone who is no longer living, this essence of who you are needs some attention. When we forget to nourish our spirit, we often find ourselves going off track—not living life as we'd like or making decisions that deviate from our values.

In this chapter we'll discuss ways to reconnect with and nourish your spirit; however, we will not discuss different religious doctrines or beliefs. Religious practices are, of course, an important way to nourish your spirit. However, given the wide array of religious beliefs, we would not be able to do justice to the topic within the scope of this book. Thus, throughout this chapter, the terms "spirit" and "spirituality" are used, especially when speaking of research focused on this topic.

WHAT DOES SPIRIT MEAN TO YOU?

You can think of spirit in many different ways: you might call it your life force, the manifestation of the divine in you, your higher power, what makes you human, or your sense of self. Spirit can also be a reflection of the interior part of yourself—the part of you where what is most dear is found, the part that gives meaning and purpose to your life, that connects you to nature, other people, animals, the stars, and everything else in the physical world. Your spirit is a source of inspiration, creativity, and strength. Spirit may feel both sacred and hard to understand, perhaps even *mystical* (having a divine meaning beyond human understanding). Take a moment now to think about how you personally define spirit.

Your Personal Definition of Spirit

In the space below, write your own personal definition of spirit or spirituality:

_____

_____

_____

_____

_____

_____

WHY IS IT IMPORTANT TO NOURISH YOUR SPIRIT?

From an integrative medicine perspective, you cannot heal the body (behaviors, physical illness) without healing the mind (thoughts and beliefs) and the spirit. In chapter 6, we discussed the connections between your behaviors, emotions, bodily sensations, core beliefs, and spirit—and how important self-expression is for your spirit. When you're not listening to your body and its cues, you may overeat, abuse your body, and develop medical problems. Being out of touch with your mind allows emotions to rage and core beliefs that no longer serve you to run your life. Disconnection from your spirit can lead to a loss of meaning and purpose, which can then lead to deep hopelessness or spirit sickness.

Indeed, hopelessness may be the most accurate sign of a spirit that is depleted or not being nourished. Research has shown that hopelessness can predict depression in cancer patients (Brothers and Andersen 2008) and is the most important predictor of the desire to commit suicide in schizophrenics (Kim, Jayathilake, and Meltzer 2003). Hopelessness has also been found to predict the development of depression and the worsening of disease in individuals with heart failure (Davidson et al. 2007), to affect the overall quality of life of patients with rheumatoid arthritis (Lu et al. 2008), and to exacerbate chronic pain conditions (Turk, Swanson, and Tunks 2008). To heal on the deepest level, it is important for body, mind, and spirit to be healed.

RESEARCH ON SPIRITUALITY AND EATING DISORDERS

Researchers have found that spirituality has a significant effect on self-esteem and quality of life in individuals seeking weight management services, and may be related to successful weight loss efforts (Popkess-Vawter, Yoder, and Gajewski 2005). People involved in spiritual programs also report reduced stress (Tuck, Alleyne, and Thinganjana 2006). In addition, one study found that individuals with eating disorders who participated in a spirituality support group during the first month of inpatient treatment improved more quickly than those in an emotional support group or a cognitive behavioral therapy group (Richards et al. 2006). Finally, obese African Americans are more likely to both respond to and adhere to faith/spirituality-based weight-loss interventions than to more secular weight-loss programs (Fitzgibbon et al. 2005; Reicks, Mills, and Henry 2004).

WAYS TO NOURISH YOUR SPIRIT

The world's main healing traditions share common principles for nourishing your spirit. These principles include gratitude, forgiveness, experiences of awe and inspiration—whether these come from nature, the birth of a baby, a sunrise, or some other way—and acceptance or unconditional love.

The Practice of Gratitude

With the possible exception of forgiveness, no practice enriches the spirit more than the practice of gratitude. In our busy working lives, so often crammed with pain or hurt, gratitude is easily forgotten. However, people who embrace gratitude as a positive way of life rather than just as something to think about during Thanksgiving may actually enjoy better health and well-being. Research has found that individuals who keep weekly gratitude journals—individuals who literally count their blessings—are more likely to exercise regularly, experience fewer negative physical symptoms, and enjoy a better quality of life. These individuals are also more likely to achieve more of their personal goals than those who are more negative or neutral about practicing gratitude, and more likely to have helped or provided emotional support to another person (Emmons and McCullough 2003). People who report being grateful also tend to report experiencing a greater number of positive emotions as well as greater optimism and satisfaction with life, and are less likely to suffer from depression and stress. This doesn't mean they deny the difficult or unpleasant aspects of life—rather, they find other aspects of their lives to be thankful for. Gratitude can also make people feel more connected with others and be more willing to be responsible for others (McCullough, Emmons, and Tsang 2002).

Sometimes when someone does something to help you, you feel you owe that person something in return. This is different from gratitude, this is *indebtedness* (the condition of owing someone something). Indebtedness tends to separate people, not bring them closer together. People who feel indebted as opposed to grateful are more likely to experience high levels of anger and fewer feelings of appreciation

(Gray, Emmons, and Morrison 2001). Being aware of and grateful for favors that others have done for you does not make you indebted.

Practicing Gratitude

Make a list of all that you are grateful for in your life:

_____

_____

_____

_____

_____

List all the ways you have shown your gratitude to others. How has showing your gratitude nourished your spirit? (Example: *I participated in the Breast Cancer Race for the Cure in memory of my best friend, Julie, who died of breast cancer. I was grateful she was in my life. Every time I look at the picture of myself at the finish line, I remember Julie and feel my spirit connecting to hers.*)

_____

_____

_____

_____

_____

List all the ways people have shown their gratitude to you. How has receiving gratitude nourished your spirit? (Example: *My coworker thanked me for helping her during a period of difficulty at work by bringing me a gift card to my favorite store. This made me feel really good.*)

_____

_____

_____

_____

_____

Forgiveness

Most moral traditions hail the ability to forgive as a virtue. Forgiveness can show up in stunning ways and in unexpected situations. We expect people who are the victims of violence or trauma to be angry; we don't expect them to forgive the perpetrator. But it happens: When a horrific shooting occurred at an Amish school in Nickel Mines, Pennsylvania in the autumn of 2006, the response of the Amish people was one of forgiveness rather than anger. Relatives of the slain children went on national media and advised forgiveness rather than hatred of the killer. Similarly, women who have been brutally raped sometimes speak of forgiving their rapist to free themselves from anger and pain. Forgiveness does not mean you condone whatever situation happened. It does not mean you were wrong and the other person was right, or that you have to pretend nothing happened. You don't have to become best friends with someone who hurt or abused you. In some ways, forgiveness is a selfish act—it's done not to make a problematic situation go away but to free you from anger and bitterness, to release the tension in your body, and allow you to move forward with your life.

Living with a sense of betrayal or a feeling that life is unfair can cause depression, physical health problems, and relationship difficulties. Being unable to forgive yourself for something you have done to another is equally damaging: this lack of self-forgiveness can lead to low self-esteem, isolation, and an inability to feel you deserve a good life. For example, if a family member has bailed you out of credit card debt related to bingeing or paid for you to get treatment, you may blame yourself for the trouble your BED/CO is putting this family member through, and have difficulty forgiving yourself. Or your eating disorder may have contributed to difficulties in your relationship with a friend. Denying yourself forgiveness on issues like these can trigger binges, increase your negative self-talk, and lower your self-esteem.

On the other hand, forgiveness has a positive effect on health and well-being. College students who are able to forgive themselves and others enjoy better physical health; self-forgiveness has an even stronger correlation with good health than forgiving others (Wilson et al. 2008). Individuals who are able to be forgiving (of themselves and others) may also have lower blood pressure and a better ability to recover from the effects of stress on the heart (Friedberg, Suchday, and Shelov 2007). Forgiveness is, moreover, also associated with less medication use, less alcohol abuse, and fewer physical symptoms (Lawler-Row et al. 2008).

Forgiveness

List people and situations by which you have felt betrayed, hurt, or mistreated; list, too, situations where you feel you have hurt another. Describe how you feel when you think of the situation now. Finally, ask yourself: Have you forgiven either the other person or yourself yet?

Situation or Person Who Has Harmed You	Situation or Person You Have Harmed	How Do You Feel When You Think of the Situation Now?	Have You Forgiven Either the Other Person or Yourself? (Forgiven/Not Forgiven)
Example: *My wife cheated on me.*		*Angry, hurt.*	*Not forgiven.*

(If you need more space, continue this part of the exercise in your journal.)

For those situations/people (including yourself) you have not yet forgiven, what effect has not forgiving this situation/person had on you? (Example: *In the case of my ex-wife, my lack of forgiveness and continuing anger have affected my ability to work successfully with her on issues related to our kids. It also makes it hard for me to trust other women I date.*)

_____

_____

_____

_____

_____

Process of forgiveness: On tiny slips of paper, write down each thing you would like to forgive others for, forgive yourself for, or be forgiven for. If you still have any emotions attached to the situation, write those down as well. Be as comprehensive as possible, giving each item its own slip of paper.

When you're finished, gather together all of your slips of paper and put them in a large fireproof container or the bottom of a barbeque—something both fireproof and deep enough to contain a fire safely. (Do this when you won't be disturbed and can be alone.) Stand or sit quietly next to the container or barbeque and, with as much compassion as possible, review in your mind the situations you've written down. For each one, say (either aloud or to yourself), "I forgive you." Allow any emotions related to the experience to surface. If you find yourself judging your emotions—or yourself for having them—say to yourself, "I forgive you for feeling _____ (emotion)." Each time you offer forgiveness, take several deep breaths. Breathe into your heart; be aware of your heartbeat and allow your heart to open and receive or dispense forgiveness.

When you have reviewed all of the situations, light the slips of paper on fire. As the slips burn, continue to affirm forgiveness for yourself and others. Do this in your own way; you might say a prayer, recite a poem, sing a song, or just state again your heartfelt forgiveness—whatever works for you. Then give yourself a hug or pat on the back: you have just done something that will change your life.

Inspiration and Awe

Inspiration is the quality of being stimulated to creative thought or activity; also, divine guidance and influence on human beings. *Awe* is a feeling of amazement mixed with respect, often coupled with a sense of personal insignificance or powerlessness. Both inspiration and awe are powerful means of nourishing the spirit. You may remember many instances in which you were inspired or felt yourself in the presence of something larger and more powerful than you. When this happens, we usually feel pretty good. But did you know that you have the ability to create these feelings for yourself?

You can and should seek opportunities to create inspiration and awe in your life. Experiences of inspiration and awe are difficult to study, so there isn't currently any research to support this, but I believe that such experiences are good not only for your spirit, but also for your health and well-being. This is in part because experiences of inspiration and awe take you out of yourself and away from your personal problems, even if just for a moment. So how do you create inspiration and awe in your life? The following are just a few of the many ways to nourish your spirit by creating—not waiting for—inspiration and a sense of awe.

READ INSPIRING BOOKS OR MAGAZINES

Books like the *Chicken Soup for the Soul* series and magazines like *Reader's Digest* and *Guideposts* offer us stories of people overcoming great hardships or finding joy in everyday things. Stories like these can often trigger inspiration.

FIND AWE IN NATURE

If you've ever spent much time around children under the age of two, you know that when you take them for a walk outside, they stop every two seconds (or so it seems) to investigate their surroundings. Everything around them inspires an ooh or an aah, whether it's a ladybug on a leaf or the blades of grass under their plump feet. Be like a child: open your heart to the mystical beauty of nature.

LISTEN TO INSPIRATIONAL RECORDINGS OR MUSIC

Sometimes listening to a specific song or piece of music can immediately shift your mood, bringing tears of happiness to your eyes. Start your day by listening to recordings or music that are uplifting and open your heart or make you want to dance. Listen on your way to work or on long car trips.

TAKE A WALK

As you walk, be aware of everything around you. Look everywhere: at the sky and the trees, at the distant horizon and the small pebbles at your feet. Listen to the sounds of the birds and the leaves rustling in the wind. Stop and smell any roses or other flowers you pass. If puppies or children are around, pause immediately to watch them and see if amusement doesn't bubble up inside of you.

CONTRIBUTE TO OTHERS

Helping others in need can inspire you, showing you the beauty and resilience of the human spirit. One year, I spent Thanksgiving volunteering at a dinner given for the homeless. I was the welcome person, greeting people who were coming in and thanking those who were leaving. In the end, I received more thank you's than I gave out. It was incredible to me that women with small children who were struggling with homelessness were able to maintain a positive spirit, at least in that moment. At the end of the day, I felt very blessed—and inspired by the human spirit.

ENJOY ART IN ALL ITS FORMS

Even if you're not an art buff, you've probably experienced a sense of awe at an art museum. Like music, art is by its very nature inspiring. Whatever your particular taste, there is some form of painting, photography, or sculpture that will inspire you. Just keep looking!

Creating Inspiration and a Sense of Awe

List activities that already inspire you or give you a sense of awe, as well as new activities you would like to try (I've listed some examples to get you started):

Visiting a historic building, museum, or church

Praying

Getting up early to take pictures of the sunrise

Bird watching

Walking along the beach or lake

Visiting an arboretum

_____

_____

_____

_____

_____

Acceptance

Soul-damaging experiences from the past can fester and eat away at your spirit. In order to shed these experiences and be free to live in the present, you must first accept your emotions, feelings, and pain. Acceptance does not mean you were not harmed. Nor does acceptance imply that your feelings are not valid and real. You can accept what happened to you without saying that it was right or good. There is a difference between having been *victimized* (meaning something happened to you or someone did something to you in the past) and being a *victim* (someone who has experienced misfortune and continues to be helpless to do anything about it). You can accept what happened to you without saying that it was right or good.

Acceptance isn't easy. It's a type of healing that requires deep soul searching—you must first be in a place in your life where you are ready to do this. You'll know when you are ready because you'll find yourself looking for solutions to the problems in your life—as you are by reading this book—rather than blaming others or justifying why you can't get on with your life. (If you're finding it difficult to move on with your life or feel numb and shut down, you may benefit from seeing a therapist.)

The first step to acceptance is making the commitment to accept what is in the past. You'll have to remind yourself of this commitment over and over again—every time your mind wants to engage in blaming, justifying, and feeling like a victim. Situations in your life that you have been unable to come to terms with may be fueling your BED/CO. For example, you may use food to soothe your feelings about a situation or your memories of it—or you may overeat to numb yourself so you won't feel out of control with emotion. When your spirit is in pain, it will cry for help and healing however it can, including by exacerbating your BED/CO.

Explore the concept of acceptance in the following exercise—try it on for size, see if you are ready to use it to nourish your soul. If you feel out of control or become very emotional, seek professional help before going any further.

Practicing Acceptance to Nourish Your Soul

Think of a situation you just can't accept: (Example: *My father divorced my mother when I was five and I never saw him again until I was an adult. I couldn't accept that he would just leave us like that—I always felt as if I had done something wrong to make him leave.*)

_____

_____

_____

_____

List three reasons why you can't accept this situation: (Example: *If I accepted this, I'd feel as if I were betraying my mother, who suffered a lot trying to raise us kids alone. I'd also feel that it made my father's actions acceptable and they're not.*)

_____

_____

_____

_____

List three ways your decision not to accept this situation (it may have been an unconscious decision) has affected your BED/CO: (Example: *I know that my bingeing gets worse when I'm in a relationship. I think it triggers all my fears of being left again.*)

_____

_____

_____

_____

Now, list three things you're afraid will happen if you accept the situation: (Example: *I'll let my guard down and I could get hurt again.*)

_____

_____

_____

_____

Finally, list three spirit-affirming thoughts you can use to refocus your attention when you find yourself engaging in soul-damaging memories from the past: (Example: *"I am healing and nourishing my spirit now more than ever."*)

_____

_____

_____

_____

Don't be hard on yourself if you find you're not ready to embrace acceptance. Acceptance requires practice. You may also need professional help to get ready.

DEVELOPING PRACTICES THAT NOURISH YOUR SPIRIT

As with any behavior change, when developing new ways to nourish your spirit, you should also put these practices on your calendar, seek support in establishing your new habits, and place reminders to yourself in visible locations (try sticky notes). Use the following exercise to establish some specific, action-oriented goals for nourishing your spirit.

Practices That Nourish Your Spirit

List specific activities you will do to nourish your spirit, as well as the date and time you will begin the activity. Remember: don't try to do everything at once. Instead, focus on a single practice for one month; then, when that practice is well-established, add a new one while continuing the first. Use the spirit-nourishing principles discussed above—gratitude, forgiveness, inspiration and awe, and acceptance—to guide your goals.

Example: *To nourish my spirit I plan to:*

1. *Keep a journal by my bed, and every night before bedtime list at least three things I'm grateful for.*

2. *Make a list of people I am not currently able to forgive but whom I would like to work on forgiving.*

3. *Go to church.*

4.   *Use acceptance techniques to practice letting go of small, everyday grievances—i.e., to stop sweating the small stuff.*

Now it's your turn! Remember: gratitude, forgiveness, inspiration and awe, and acceptance.

_____

_____

_____

_____

_____

_____

SUMMARY

When you nourish your spirit by filling yourself up with the good feelings of gratitude, forgiveness, awe, and acceptance, you are more able to give to others. Many of you may have spent your life draining your spiritual well through taking care of others at the expense of yourself. This lack of spiritual nurturance can fuel emotionally driven bingeing. You may also overeat as a way to fill up your spirit, turning to food instead of practices like forgiveness and gratitude. Long-held regrets, a lack of acceptance, and a lack of forgiveness can leave you exhausted and depressed, further exacerbating your BED/CO. When you take care of your spirit, you will have much more to offer other people and it will come from a place of abundance rather than indebtedness, guilt, or obligation. Take some time every day—even if only five minutes—to nourish your spirit. You won't regret it.

Conclusion: Five Steps to Healing from Eating Disorders

It is my sincere hope that this book has been a significant and helpful part of your recovery from binge eating disorder or compulsive overeating. In this final section we will discuss five steps you can take to keep moving forward in your recovery. These five steps will empower you to take charge of your life, so that you continue to heal in body, mind, and spirit.

STEP 1: PUT YOUR ATTENTION ON YOUR HEALTH FIRST

Throughout this book, we've discussed the pitfalls of placing too much of your attention on your weight, emotions, and past experiences. Where you place your attention is where you will achieve the most positive—and negative—results. To support your recovery, place your attention squarely on creating good health for yourself. With every decision you make, ask yourself, "Will this contribute to my good health?" Consider its impact on nutrition, exercise, emotional regulation, medical concerns, body image concerns, and so on.

When your attention is on your health, over time you will make better choices about what and how much to eat, enjoy and appreciate your body more, and be more physically active. In the following exercise, list steps you would like to take/areas you want to attend to over the next three months to improve and support good health in mind, body, and spirit.

What You Will Do to Improve and Support Good Health

Steps you will take to improve your mental health: (Example: *Make an appointment with a therapist; take supplements to support my mood; practice meditating every morning before work for five minutes.*)

_____

_____

_____

_____

_____

Steps you will take to improve your physical health: (Example: *Walk fifteen minutes a day, five days a week; make an appointment for a complete physical exam; eat at least three vegetables every day.*)

_____

_____

_____

_____

_____

Steps you will take to improve your spiritual health: (Example: *Stop judging myself; start a gratitude journal; share my true feelings, when appropriate, with those I'm in relationships with; do something fun every single week.*)

_____

_____

_____

_____

_____

List new steps—or goals—for good health every three months. If you're able to establish more long-term objectives, also set goals for one year from now and even five years from now.

To-Do List for Three-Month Goals

Whether your goal is long-term or short-term, it's a good idea to first make a list of whatever you need to do in order to achieve the goal. For example, if your goal is to start a walking program, your to-do list might include purchasing sturdy walking shoes and socks, identifying a safe walking path, and calling a friend to see if she will walk with you. List the activities you need to do now in order to accomplish your three-month goals (the goals or steps you outlined in the previous exercise):

Goal: _____

To-do list: _____

_____

_____

_____

Goal: _____

To-do list: _____

_____

_____

_____

Goal: _____

To-do list: _____

_____

_____

_____

(If you need more space, continue this exercise in your journal.)

Finally, add these to-do list activities to your calendar. Scheduling them is an important step to getting them done. Get your calendar out right now and do this.

STEP 2: EXPLORE THE MANY ROADS TO HEALING

Over the course of this book, we've discussed many different tools you can use to facilitate your journey to healing. Use these tools to create a master treatment plan that addresses all of the obstacles you personally face. In the following exercise, write down the particular therapies, supplements, doctors, or other providers you want to try. Be as specific as you can.

Your Individual Master Treatment Plan

Your plan for stress reduction: (Example: *I'll schedule a massage for twice a month. I'll also reread the chapter on stress tools and decide which supplements to take.*)

_____

_____

_____

_____

_____

Your plan for addressing medical or psychological issues: (Example: *I'll consult an acupuncturist about my insomnia and try valerian.*)

_____

_____

_____

_____

_____

Your plan for working on your nutrition: (Example: *I'll eat more fresh fruits and vegetables; I'll take a multivitamin every day.*)

_____

_____

_____

_____

_____

Other issues you would like to target and your plan for working on them:

_____

_____

_____

_____

_____

The most important thing to remember is that if something doesn't work for you, try something else—but keep trying! (Note that typically you'll need to take a supplement for at least a month to determine if it works for you.) And be creative—investigate other ways of achieving your goals. I strongly recommend that you incorporate the use of complementary and alternative therapies into your master treatment plan. You may be surprised by the benefits you reap. Whatever you do, don't give up.

STEP 3: KEEP YOUR WORD TO YOURSELF

How many times have you made an important promise to yourself only to break it soon afterward? You may be very good at keeping your promises to other people but not so good at keeping your promises to yourself. I know many mothers who would die before they'd break a promise to their child but yet regularly break promises to themselves.

Keeping your word to yourself requires practice. Don't be hard on yourself if you find it difficult at first. The key is to start with small things. Can you keep your promise to yourself to take a multivitamin every day, or to take your prescription medication as directed? Keeping promises to yourself is like building a muscle: your ability to do it grows stronger the more you use it.

If you are unable to keep your promises to yourself, ask yourself why. Was the promise unrealistic? Was there some obstacle to fulfilling it? If you find yourself making excuses for not keeping your promise, look for ways to eliminate even the possibility of an excuse. For example, if you forgot the promise, put sticky notes all over your house or ask everyone at home or work to support you by reminding you of your promise.

In the following exercise, list three promises to yourself you would like to keep. Focus on one promise a week. The following week, choose another promise to focus on, and so on. Repeat the cycle for three months. Once you've mastered the first three promises, go on to three more, and then three more. Remember: where there's a will, there's a way.

Three Promises to Yourself You Will Keep During the Next Three Months

Your promises to yourself from _____ (date) to _____ (date):

1. _____

2. _____

3. _____

Describe how it feels to keep promises to yourself:

_____

_____

_____

STEP 4: IN ALL THINGS, CHOOSE THE THOUGHT OR ACTION THAT MAKES YOU FEEL THE MOST WHOLE

You may be in the habit of doing things to please others whether or not it makes you feel good—maybe even things that actually hurt you mentally, physically, or spiritually. To choose the thought or action that makes *you* feel most whole, you have to first respect and value yourself. This can be difficult if you have BED/CO, because past experiences may have depleted your spirit or lowered your self-esteem. That's okay: the practice of appreciating yourself will fill up the empty well left by past experiences. So even if you don't believe right now that you are worth loving, act as if you do and one day you will.

Choosing the thought or action that makes you feel most whole requires using both brain power and body power. When you make a decision, see how it feels to your body. Do you feel a sense of wise resonance? If so, this is the right action. If your body is uncomfortable—you feel physical discomfort—but your mind keeps making excuses, reexamine your decision.

If you find yourself justifying staying in a relationship with someone who does not meet your needs, see if you can get help to address your concerns about the relationship. Changing your perceptions of, and responses to, your partner's behavior may not end the relationship as you fear—it may make it better. No matter what happens, you will have taken action to make yourself feel whole.

Choosing the Action That Makes You Feel Whole

List current or past situations in which you either did something that was not in your best interest, or allowed yourself to be hurt: (Example: *I stayed in an abusive relationship; I let my boss bully me; I volunteered for a committee at church when I knew I was too busy.*)

_____

_____

_____

_____

_____

Next, make a list of the things that make you feel whole; include on this list the qualities you value in yourself: (Example: *I feel whole when I am told the truth, appreciated, and treated with respect. I value my ability to be honest, kind, and generous. I am a person who is both lovable and loving.*)

_____

_____

_____

_____

_____

Put this list somewhere prominent to remind yourself daily of who you are and what makes you feel whole.

STEP 5: DON'T TRY TO DO IT ALONE—ASK FOR SUPPORT

If you have BED/CO, you may be reluctant to ask for help. You may pride yourself on taking care of other people, and yet feel empty and lonely yourself. Know that you can't continually give to others if you don't nurture yourself physically, mentally, and spiritually. Asking for support can help reduce stress, build relationships, and break the cycle of being expected to be able to do it all.

Support can come from a variety of sources, including support groups, health care professionals, and family and friends. For example, groups such as Overeaters Anonymous (OA) and Eating Disorders Anonymous (EDA) can help support you in your recovery. If you have medical concerns or problems you can't handle, seek support from a health care professional. Personal coaching can be another excellent source of support. And as we've discussed, it's important to build a network of supportive individuals you can turn to in times of need. Remember, though, support isn't a one-way street: supporting others without ever asking for support yourself won't help you.

If you've historically tried to do everything yourself, people may also have come to expect this behavior from you; when given extra work, you may have to say no. If you're in a work group or family that isn't used to carrying their own weight—perhaps because you've done it for them in the past— you'll have to set up some boundaries; for example, you might say, "I'll wash the dishes if you'll wipe the counters and put away the food."

Don't expect people to be able to read your mind or know intuitively what you need to feel supported. Tell them explicitly what you need—and then allow them to give it to you. And don't expect everyone to be happy with the changes. When you start setting boundaries, you're likely to hear some grumbling. Don't let that stop you. Your goal is to continue to focus on your recovery. Getting support is part of what it takes to heal from BED/CO; support impacts all areas of your health and well-being, including your recovery. So, go ahead—reach out and lean on someone else for a bit. You'll feel much stronger for it.

Your Plan for Asking for Support

What, specifically, makes you feel supported? (Example: *I feel supported when I share my responsibilities and am part of a strong team. I feel supported when people show their gratitude for something I've done instead of taking me for granted.*)

_____

_____

_____

_____

_____

What actions can you take to get the support you need? (Example: *I can ask my husband to take care of the kids while I go to the gym.*)

_____

_____

_____

_____

_____

_____

In order to make this more concrete, use your journal to lay out a timeline for the specific actions you plan to take to obtain the support you need.

SUMMARY

This book was designed to empower you to take charge of your life and overcome your bingeing or compulsive overeating. By working through the exercises in this book, you have committed yourself to your recovery. This commitment will give you the momentum to bring your dreams of transforming your life to fruition. Don't be afraid. Continue to focus your attention on recovery. Continue to recommit, even when the odds seem to be against you or it feels like you're taking three steps backward for every two steps forward. Sometimes the journey to recovery isn't clear; however, by harnessing the power of your commitment and intention, you will get there.

For all of you who've taken the time to read the words set down in this book, I offer my sincere gratitude and appreciation. May you be blessed with the miracle of recovery!

—Carolyn Coker Ross, MD, MPH

Resources

For more information about complementary and alternative therapies, supplements, and herbs for BED/CO, visit my website at: www.carolynrossmd.com.

The following are other resources that you may find useful. Please use your own good sense when choosing practitioners and therapists through any means. I am not endorsing the following resources by listing them here.

NUTRITION

Centers for Disease Control and Prevention—provides further information about nutrition: www.cdc.gov/nccdphp/dnpa/nutrition/nutrition_for_everyone/basics.

The Glycemic Index—provides further information on glycemic loads: www.glycemicindex.com.

The U.S. Department of Agriculture—offers an online meal-tracking system: www.mypyramidtracker.gov/planner.

TRADITIONAL APPROACHES TO TREATING BED/CO

Behavioral Tech LLC—offers a directory of dialectical behavioral therapists: www.behavioraltech.org.

The National Association of Cognitive-Behavioral Therapists—offers information about cognitive behavioral therapy (CBT) as well as a directory of certified CBT therapists: www.nacbt.org.

HEALING THERAPIES FOR STRESS MANAGEMENT

American Chiropractic Association—offers information about chiropractic as well as a directory of chiropractors: www.amerchiro.org.

American Massage Therapy Association—offers information about massage as well as a directory of massage therapists: www.amtamassage.org.

National Certification Commission for Acupuncture and Oriental Medicine—offers a directory of acupuncturists: www.nccaom.org.

The Reiki Alliance—offers information about reiki (a type of energy medicine) as well as a directory of practitioners: www.reikialliance.com.

Zero Balancing Health Association—offers information about Zero Balancing (a type of energy medicine) as well as a directory of practitioners: www.zerobalancing.com.

MINDFULNESS

Nhat Hahn, T. 1999. *The Miracle of Mindfulness: An Introduction to the Practice of Meditation.* Boston: Beacon Press.

References

Albu, J. B., L. Murphy, D. H. Frager, J. A. Johnson, and F. X. Pi-Sunyer. 1997. Visceral fat and race dependent health risks in obese nondiabetic premenopausal women. *Diabetes* 46:456–462.

Allender, P. S., J. A. Cutler, D. Follmann, F. P. Cappuccio, J. Pryer, and P. Elliott. 1996. Dietary calcium and blood pressure. *Annals of Internal Medicine* 124:825–831.

Allison, K. C., C. M. Grilo, R. M. Masheb, and A. J. Stunkard. 2007. High self-reported rates of neglect and emotional abuse, by persons with binge eating disorder and night eating syndrome. *Behaviour Research and Therapy* 45(12):2874–2883.

American Institute of Cancer Research. 2001. Impact of 9-11 attacks on American diet and lifestyle. www.icrsurvey.com/Study.aspx?f=AICR_0802.html. Accessed January 19, 2009.

American Psychiatric Association. 2000. *Diagnostic and Statistical Manual of Mental Disorders*, fourth edition, text revision. Washington D.C.: American Psychiatric Association.

American Psychiatric Association. 2006. *Practice Guidelines for the Treatment of Patients with Eating Disorders*, third edition. Washington D.C.: American Psychiatric Association.

Anbar, R., and A. Savedoff. 2005. Treatment of binge eating with automatic word processing and self-hypnosis: A case report. *The American Journal of Clinical Hypnosis* 48:191–198.

Andreatini, R., V. Sartori, M. Seabra, and J. Leite. 2002. Effect of valepotriates (valerian extract) in generalized anxiety disorder: A randomized placebo-controlled pilot study. *Phytotherapy Research* 16:650–654.

Andrews, B. 1995. Bodily shame as a mediator between abusive experiences and depression. *Journal of Abnormal Psychology* 104:277–285.

Appolinario, J., A. Godoy-Mato, L. Fontenelle, L. Carraro, M. Cabral, A. Viera, and W. Coutinho. 2002. An open-label trial of sibutramine in obese patients with binge eating disorder. *Journal of Clinical Psychiatry* 63:28–30.

Appolinario, J. C., and S. L. McElroy. 2004. Pharmacological approaches in the treatment of binge eating disorder. *Current Drug Targets* 5(3):301–307.

Armas, L. A. G., B. W. Hollis, and R. P. Heaney. 2004. Vitamin D2 is much less effective than vitamin D3 in humans. *Journal of Clinical Endocrinology and Metabolism* 89:5387–5391.

Aro, A., S. Mannisto, I. Salminen, M. L. Ovaskainen, V. Kataja, and M. Uusitupa. 2000. Inverse association between dietary and serum conjugated linoleic acid and risk of breast cancer in postmenopausal women. *Nutrition and Cancer* 38(2):151–157.

Aronson, W. J., J. A. Glaspy, S. T. Reddy, D. Reese, D. Heber, and D. Bagga. 2001. Modulation of omega-3/omega-6 polyunsaturated ratios with dietary fish oils in men with prostate cancer. *Urology* 58:283–288

Autier, P., and S. Gandini. 2007. Vitamin D supplementation and total mortality: A meta-analysis of randomized controlled trials. *Archives of Internal Medicine* 167:1730–1737.

Babyak, M., J. A. Blumenthal, S. Herman, P. Khatri, M Doraiswamy, K. Moore, W. E. Craighead, T. T. Baldewicz, and K. R. Krishnan. 2000. Exercise treatment for major depression: Maintenance of therapeutic benefit at 10 months. *Psychosomatic Medicine* 62(5):633–638.

Bacon, L., N. L. Keim, M. D. Van Loan, M. Derricote, B. Gale, and A. Kazaks. 2002. Evaluating a "non-diet" wellness intervention for improvement of metabolic fitness, psychological well-being, and eating and activity behaviors. *International Journal of Obesity Related Metabolic Disorders* 26(6):854–865.

Bannerman, R. H. 1979. Acupuncture: The WHO view. World Health Organization.

Barringer, T.A., J. K. Kirk, A. C. Santaniello, K. L. Foley, and R. Michielutte. 2003. Effect of a multivitamin and mineral supplement on infection and quality of life: A randomized, double-blind, placebo-controlled trial. *Annals of Internal Medicine* 138:365–371.

Barlow, C. E., H. W. Kohl III, L. W. Gibbons, and S. N. Blair. 1995. Physical fitness, mortality, and obesity. *International Journal of Obesity* 19:S41–S44.

Bell, C., L. Adair, and B. Popkin. 2003. Ethnic differences in the association between BMI and Hypertension. *American Journal of Epidemiology* 155:346–353.

Bertone-Johnson, E. R., S. E. Hankinson, A. Bendich, S. R. Johnson, W. C. Willett, and J. E. Manson. 2005. Calcium and vitamin D intake and risk of incident premenstrual syndrome. *Archives of Internal Medicine.* 165(11):1246–1252.

Blair, S., and S. Brodney. 1999. Effects of physical inactivity and obesity on morbidity and mortality: Current evidence and research issues. *Medicine and Science in Sports and Exercise* 31: S646–S662.

Boggiano, M. M., A. I. Artiga, C. E. Pritchett, P. C. Chandler-Laney, M. L. Smith, and A. J. Eldridge. 2007. High intake of palatable foods predicts binge eating independent of susceptibility to obesity: An animal model of lean vs. obese binge eating and obesity with and without binge-eating. *International Journal of Obesity* 31:1357–1367.

Bowers, W. 1990. Treatment of depressed in-patients: Cognitive therapy plus medication, relaxation plus medication, and medication alone. *British Journal of Psychiatry* 156:73–78.

Bray, G. A., S. J. Nielsen, and B. M. Popkin. 2004. Consumption of high-fructose corn syrup in beverages may play a role in the epidemic of obesity. *American Journal of Clinical Nutrition* 79(4):537–543.

Breslow, J. L. 2006. N-3 fatty acids and cardiovascular disease. *American Journal of Clinical Nutrition.* 83(6S):1477S–1482S.

Briazgounov, I. P. 1988. The role of physical activity in the prevention and treatment of noncommunicable diseases. *World Health Statistics Quarterly* 41:242–250.

Brownell, K. D., and J. Rodin. 1994. Medical, metabolic, and psychological effects of weight cycling. *Archives Internal Medicine* 154:1325–1330.

Brownley, K., N. Berkman, J. Sedway, K. Lohr, and C. Bulik. 2007. Binge eating disorder treatment: A systematic review of randomized controlled trials. *International Journal of Eating Disorders* 40:337–348.

Brothers, B., and B. Andersen. 2008. Hopelessness as a predictor of depressive symptoms for breast cancer patients coping with recurrence. *Psycho-Oncology.* www.ncbi.nlm.nih.gov/pubmed/18702065. Accessed January 16, 2009.

Bruinsma, K. A., and D. L. Taren. 2000. Dieting, essential fatty acid intake, and depression. *Nutrition Reviews* 58:98–108.

Cangiano, C., F. Ceci, A. Cascino, M. Del Ben, A. Laviano, M. Muscaritoli, F. Antonucci, and F. Rossi-Fanelli. 1992. Eating behavior and adherence to dietary prescriptions in obese adult subjects treated with 5-hydroxytryptophan. *American Journal of Clinical Nutrition* 56:863–867.

Carlson, L., M. Speca, K. Patel, and E. Goodey. 2004. Mindfulness-based stress reduction in relation to quality of life, mood, symptoms of stress, and levels of cortisol, dehydroepiandrosterone sulfate (DHEAS), and melatonin in breast and prostate cancer outpatients. *Psychoneuroendocrinology* 29:448–474.

Castellini, G., F. Lapi, C. Ravaldi, A. Vannacci, C. M. Rotella, C. Faravelli, and V. Ricca. 2008. Eating disorder psychopathology does not predict the overweight severity in subjects seeking weight loss treatment. *Comparative Psychiatry* 49:359–363.

Centers for Disease Control. 2002. 2001 BRFSS summary data quality report. Atlanta, GA: U.S. Department of Health and Human Services, CDC.

Chan, J., M. Stampfer, J. Ma, P. Gann, M. Gaziano, and E. Giovannucci. 2001. Dairy products, calcium, and prostate cancer risk in the Physicians Health Study. *American Journal of Clinical Nutrition* 74:549–554.

Chen, E., L. Matthews, C. Allen, J. Kuo, and M. M. Linehan. 2008. Dialectical behavior therapy for clients with binge eating disorder or bulimia nervosa and borderline personality disorder. *International Journal of Eating Disorders* 41:505–512

Choi, S. 1999. Vitamin B12 deficiency: A new risk factor for breast cancer? *Nutrition Reviews* 57: 250–260.

Claes, S. 2004a. Corticotropin-releasing hormone (CRH) in psychiatry: From stress to psychopathology. *Annals of Medicine* 36:50–61.

———. 2004b. CRH, stress, and major depression: A psychobiological interplay. *Vitamins and Hormones* 69:117–150.

Cleland, L. G., G. E. Caughey, M. J. James, and S. M. Proudman. 2006. Reduction of cardiovascular risk factors with long-term fish oil treatment in early rheumatoid arthritis. *Journal of Rheumatology* 33:1973–1979.

Colin, A, J. Reggers, and V. Castronovo. 2003. Lipids, depression, and suicide. *Encephale* 29:49–58.

Coppen, A., and J. Bailey. 2000. Enhancement of the antidepressant action of fluoxetine by folic acid: A randomised, placebo controlled trial. *Journal of Affective Disorders* 60:121–131.

Coppen, A., P. C. Whybrow, R. Noguera, R. Maggs, and A. J. Prange. 1972. The comparative antidepressant value of L-tryptophan and imipramine with and without attempted potentiation by liothyronine. *Archives of General Psychiatry* 26:234–241.

Cumming, R., P. Mitchell, and W. Smith. 2000. Diet and cataract: The Blue Mountains Eye Study. *Ophthalmology* 10:450–456.

Dallman, M., N. Pecoraro, S. Akana, S. La Fleur, F. Gomez, H. Houshyar, M. E. Bell, S. Bhatnagar, K. Laugero, and S. Manalo. 2003. Chronic stress and obesity: A new view of "comfort food." *Proceedings of the National Academy of Science* 100:11696–11701.

Davidson, J. and K. Connor. 2001. St. John's Wort in generalized anxiety disorder: Three case reports. *Journal of Clinical Psychopharmacology* 21:635–636.

Davidson, P., K. Dracup, J. Phillips, J. Daly, and G. Padilla. 2007. Preparing for the worst while hoping for the best: The relevance of hope in the heart failure illness trajectory. *Journal of Cardiovascular Nursing* 22:159–165.

Davidson, R., J. Kabat-Zinn, J. Schumacher, M. Rosenkranz, D. Muller, S. Santorelli, F. Urbanowski, A. Harrington, K. Bonus, and J. Sheridan. 2003. Alterations in brain and immune function produced by mindfulness meditation. *Psychosomatic Medicine* 65:564–570.

De Deckere, E. A. M. 1999. Possible beneficial effect of fish and fish n-3 polyunsaturated fatty acids in breast and colorectal cancer. *European Journal of Cancer Prevention* 8:213–221.

Delle, R., P. Pancheri, and P. Scapicchio. 2002. Efficacy and tolerability of oral and intramuscular S-adenosyl-L-methionine 1,4-butanedisulfonate (SAMe) in the treatment of major depression: Comparison with imipramine in two multicenter studies. *American Journal of Clinical Nutrition* 76:1172S–1176S.

Deutch, B. 1995. Menstrual pain in Danish women correlated with low n-3 polyunsaturated fatty acid intake. *European Journal of Clinical Nutrition* 49:508–516.

Diaz, A., and R. Motta. 2008. The effects of an aerobic exercise program on post-traumatic stress disorder symptom severity in adolescents. *International Journal of Emerging Mental Health* 10:49–59.

Dichi, I., P. Frenhane, J. B. Dichi, C. R. Correa, A. Y. Angeleli, and M. H. Bicudo. 2000. Comparison of omega-3 fatty acids and sulfasalazine in ulcerative colitis. *Nutrition* 16:87–90.

Dobie D. J., D. R. Kivlahan, C. Maynard, K. R. Bush, T. M. Davis, K. A. Bradley. 2004. Posttraumatic stress disorder in female veterans: Association with self-reported health problems and functional impairment. *Archives of Internal Medicine*. 164(4): 394-400.

Donath, F., S. Quispe, K. Diefenbach, A. Maurer, and I. Fietze. 2000. Roots I: Critical evaluation of the effect of valerian extract on sleep structure and sleep quality. *Pharmacopsychiatry* 33:47–53

Drenowski, A, D. D. Krahn, M. A., Demitrack, K. Nairn, and B. A. Gosnell. 1995. Naloxone, an opiate blocker, reduces the consumption of sweet high-fat foods in obese and lean female binge eaters. *The American Journal of Clinical Nutrition* 61(6):1206–1212.

Ebbesson, S. O., P. M. Risica, L. O. Ebbesson, J. M. Kennish, and M. E. Tejero. 2005. Omega-3 fatty acids improve glucose tolerance and components of the metabolic syndrome in Alaskan Eskimos: The Alaska Siberia Project. *International Journal of Circumpolar Health* 64:396–408.

Emmons. R. A., and M. E. McCullough. 2003. Counting blessings versus burdens: Experimental studies of gratitude and subjective well-being in daily life. *Journal of Personality and Social Psychology* 84:377–389.

Esplen, M. F., P. E. Garfinkel, M. Olmsted, R. M. Gallop, and S. Kennedy. 1998. A randomized controlled trial of guided imagery in bulimia nervosa. *Psychological Medicine* 28:1347–1357.

Fabricatore, A. N., and T. A. Wadden. 2003. Psychological functioning of obese individuals. *Diabetes Spectrum* 16(4):245–252.

Fairburn, C. G., H. A. Doll, S. L. Welch, P. J. Hay, B. A. Davies, and M. E. O'Connor. 1998. Risk factors for binge eating disorder. *Archives of General Psychiatry* 55:425–432.

Field, A., L. Cheung, A. Wolf, D. Herzog, S. Gortmaker, and G. Colditz. 1999. Exposure to the mass media and weight concerns among girls. *Pediatrics* 103(3):e36.

Field, T., C. Morrow, C. Valdeon, S. Larson, C. Kuhn, and S. Schanberg. 1992. Massage reduces anxiety in child and adolescent psychiatric patients. *Journal of American Academy of Child and Adolescent Psychiatry* 31(1):125–131.

Field, T., M. Hernandez-Reif, M. Diego, S. Schanberg, and C. Kuhn. 2005. Cortisol decreases and serotonin and dopamine increases following massage therapy. *International Journal of Neuroscience* 115:1397–1413.

Field, T., A. Martinez, T. Nawrocki, J. Pickens, N. A. Fox, and S. Schanberg. 1998. Music shifts frontal EEG in depressed adolescents. *Adolescence* 33:109–116.

Field, T., S. Schanberg, C. Kuhn, T. Field T, K. Fieero, T. Henteleff, C. Mueller, R. Yando, S. Shaw, and I. Burman. 1998. Bulimic adolescents benefit from massage therapy. *Adolescence* 33:555–563.

Field, T., S. Seligman, F. Scalfidi, and S. Schanberg. 1996. Alleviating post-traumatic stress in children following Hurricane Andrew. *Journal of Applied Development Psychology* 17:37–50.

Firk, C., and C. R. Marksu. 2007. Review: Serotonin by stress interaction: A susceptibility factor for the development of depression? *Journal of Psychopharmacology* 21:538–544.

Fitzgibbon, M., M. Stolley, P. Ganschow, L. Schiffer, A. Wells, N. Simon, and A. Dyer. 2005. Results of a faith-based weight loss intervention for black women. *Journal of the National Medical Association* 97:1393–1402.

Fleshner, M. 2005. Physical activity and stress resistance: Sympathetic nervous system adaptations prevent stress-induced immunosuppression. *Exercise Sport Sciences Reviews* 33:120–126.

Fontaine, K., D. Redden, C. Wang, A. Westfall, and D. Allison. 2003. Years of life lost due to obesity. *Journal of the American Medical Association* 289:187–193.

Foster-Powell, K., S. Holt, and J. C. Brand-Miller. 2002. International table of glycemic index and glycemic load values. *American Journal of Clinical Nutrition* 76:5–56

Friedberg, J., S. Suchday, and D. Shelov. 2007. The impact of forgiveness on cardiovascular reactivity and recovery. *International Journal of Psychophysiology* 65:87–94.

Gadde, K. M., K. R. R. Krishnan, and M. K. Drezner. 1997. Bupropion SR shows promise as an effective obesity treatment. *Obesity Research* 7(1):S51.

Garland, C. F., F. C. Garland, and E. D. Gorham. 2006. The role of vitamin D in cancer prevention. *American Journal of Public Health* 96:252–261.

Gilbert, P., J. Pehl, and S. Allan. 1994. The phenomenology of shame and guilt: An empirical investigation. *British Journal of Medical Psychology* 67: 23–36.

Gillman, M. W., L. A. Cupples, D. Gagnon, B. M. Posner, R. C. Ellison, W. P. Castelli, and P. A. Wolf. 1995. Protective effects of fruits and vegetables on development of stroke in men. *Journal of the American Medical Association* 273:1113-1117.

Gluck, M., A. Geliebter, and M. Lorence. 2004. Cortisol stress response is positively correlated with central obesity in obese women with binge eating disorder (BED) before and after cognitive-behavioral treatment. *Annals of the New York Academy of Science* 2032:202–207.

Goldfein, J. A., B. T. Walsh, J. L. LaChauseé, H. R. Kissileff, and M. J. Devlin. 1993. Eating behavior in binge eating disorder. *International Journal of Eating Disorders* 14: 427–431.

Gray, S. A., R. A. Emmons, and A. Morrison. 2001. Distinguishing gratitude from indebtedness in affect and action tendencies. Poster presented at the annual meeting of the American Psychological Association, San Francisco, CA.

Greenwood, B., and M. Fleshner. 2008. Exercise, learned helplessness, and the stress-resistant brain. *Neuromolecular Medicine* 10:81–98.

Greist, J. H., M. H. Klein, R. R. Eischens, J. Faris, A. S. Gurman, and W. P. Morgan. 1978. Running through your mind. *Journal of Psychosomatic Research* 22:259–294.

Grilo, C, R. Masheb, M. Bordy, C. Toth, C. Burke-Martindale, and B. Rothschild. 2005. Childhood maltreatment in extremely obese male and female bariatric surgery candidates. *Obesity Research* 13(1):123–130.

Grucza, R., T. Przybeck, and R. Cloninger. 2007. Prevalence and correlates of binge eating disorder in a community sample *Comparative Psychiatry* 48:124–131.

Guizhen, L., Z. Yunjun, G. Linxiang, and L. Aizhen. 1998. Comparative study on acupuncture combined with behavioral desensitization for treatment of anxiety neuroses. *American Journal of Acupuncutre* 26(2-3):117–120.

Guss, J. L., H. R. Kissilef, B. T. Walsh, and M. J. Devlin. 1994. Binge eating behavior in patients with eating disorders. *Obesity Research* 2(4):355–363.

Han, J. S. 1986. Electroacupuncture: An alternative to antidepressants for treating affective diseases? *International Journal of Neuroscience* 29(1–2):79–92.

Hart, S., T. Field, M. Hernandez-Reif, G. Nearing, S. Shaw, S. Schanberg, and C. Kuhn. 2001. Anorexia nervosa symptoms are reduced by massage therapy. *Eating Disorders* 9:289–299.

He, K., E. Rimm, and A. Merchant. 2002. Fish consumption and risk of stroke in men. *The Journal of the American Medical Association* 288:3130–3136.

Hollifield, M., N. Sinclair-Lian, T. Warner, and R. Hammerschlag. 2007. Acupuncture for post-traumatic stress disorder: A randomized controlled pilot trial. *Journal of Nervous and Mental Diseases* 195(6):504–513.

Holman, R. T., C. E. Adams, and R. A. Nelson. 1995. Patients with anorexia nervosa demonstrate deficiencies of selected essential fatty acids, compensatory changes inonessential fatty acids, and decreased fluidity of plasma lipids. *Journal of Nutrition* 125:901–907.

Holmes, T., and R. Rahe. 1967. Holmes-Rahe social readjustment rating scale. *Journal of Psychosomatic Research* 2:214.

Hu, F., and E. Cho. 2003. Fish and long-chain omega-3 fatty acid intake and risk of coronary heart disease and total mortality in diabetic women. *Circulation* 107:1852–1857.

Hu, F. and M. Stampfer. 1999. Nut consumption and risk of coronary heart disease: A review of epidemiologic evidence. *Current Atherosclerosis Reports* 1:204–209.

Huff, J., and J. LaDou. 2007. Aspartame bioassay findings portend human cancer hazards. *International Journal of Occupational Environmental Health* 13:446–448.

Hutto, B. R. 1997. Folate and cobalamin in psychiatric illness. *Comprehensive Psychiatry* 38:305–14.

Institute of Medicine (Food and Nutrition Board). 1998. *Dietary Reference Intakes: Thiamin, Riboflavin, Niacin, Vitamin B6, Folate, Vitamin B12, Pantothenic Acid, Biotin, and Choline*. Washington, D.C.: National Academy Press.

Janakiramaiah, N., B. N. Gangadhar, P. J. Naga Venkatesha Murthy, M. G. Harish, D. K. Subbakrishna, and A. Vedamurthachar. 2000. Antidepressant efficacy of Sudarshan Kriya Yoga (SKY) in melancholia: A randomized comparison with electroconvulsive therapy and imipramine. *Journal of Affective Disorders* 57:255–257.

Javaras, K. N., N. M. Laird, T. Reichborn-Kjennerud, C. M. Bulik, H. G. Pope, and J. I. Hudson. 2008. Familiality and heritability of binge eating disorder: Results of a case-control family study and a twin study. *International Journal of Eating Disorders* 41(2):174–179.

Javaras, K. N., H. G. Pope, J. K. Lalonde, J. L. Roberts, Y. I. Nillni, N. M. Laird, C. M. Bulik, S. J. Crow, S. L. McElroy, B. T. Walsh, M. T. Tsuang, N. R. Rosenthal, and J. I. Hudson. 2008.

Co-occurrence of binge eating disorder with psychiatric and medical disorders. *Journal of Clinical Psychiatry* 69(2):266–273.

Jennings, E. 1995. Folic acid as a cancer preventing agent. *Medical Hypothesis* 45:297–303.

Jiang, R., J. Manson, M. Stampfer, S. Liu, W. Willett, and F. Hu. 2002. Nut and peanut butter consumption and risk of type 2 diabetes in women. *Journal of the American Medical Association* 288:2554–2560.

Johnsen, L., A. Gorin, A. Stone, and D. le Grange. 2003. Characteristics of binge eating among women in the community seeking treatment for binge eating or weight loss. *Eating Behaviors* 3:295–305.

Johnson, J. G., P. Cohen, S. Kasen, and J. S. Brook. 2006. Personality disorder traits evident by early adulthood and risk for eating and weight problems during middle adulthood. *International Journal of Eating Disorders* 39(3):184–192.

Jonas, W. B., C. P. Rapoza, and W. F. Blair. 1996. The effect of niacinamide on osteoarthritis: A pilot study. *Inflammatory Research* 45:330–334.

Jones, N. A., and T. Field. 1999. Massage and music therapies attenuate frontal EEG asymmetry in depressed adolescents. *Adolescence* 34(135):529–34.

Kahn, R. S., H. G. Westenberg, and W. M. Verhoeven. 1987. Effect of a serotonin precursor and uptake inhibitor in anxiety disorders: A double-blind comparison of 5-hydroxytryptophan, clomipramine, and placebo. *International Clinical Psychopharmacology* 2:33–45.

Kahn, R. S., and H. G. M. Westenberg. 1985. L-5-hydroxytryptophan in the treatment of anxiety disorders. *Journal of Affective Disorders* 8:197–200.

Kajander, K., K. Hatakka, and T. Poussa. 2005. A probiotic mixture alleviates symptoms in irritable bowel syndrome patients: A controlled 6-month intervention. *Alimentary Pharmacology and Therapeutics* 22:387–394.

Kampman, M., T. Wilsgaard, and S. Mellgren. 2007. Outdoor activities and diet in childhood and adolescence relate to MS risk above the Arctic Circle. *Journal of Neurology* 254(4):471–477.

Kampman, E., M. L. Slattery, B. Caan, and J. D. Potter. 2000. Calcium, vitamin D, sunshine exposure, dairy products, and colon cancer risk. *Cancer Causes Control* 11:459–466

Keel, P., D. Dorer, D. Franko, S. Jackson, and D. Herzog. 2005. Post-remission predictors of relapse in women with eating disorders. *American Journal of Psychiatry* 162:2263–2268.

Keel, P. K. 2005. *Eating Disorders*. Upper Saddle River, N.J.: Pearson/Prentice Hall.

Kim, C., K. Jayathilake, and H. Meltzer. 2003. Hopelessness, neurocognitive function, and insight in schizophrenia: Relationship to suicidal behavior. *Schizophrenia Research* 60:71–80.

Kimmons, J. E., H. M. Blanck, B. C. Tohill, J. Zhang, and L. K. Khan. 2006. Multivitamin use in relation to self-reported body mass index and weight loss attempts. *Medscape General Medicine* 8(3):3.

Kirsch, I., G. Montgomery, and G. Sapirstein. 1995. Hypnosis as an adjunct to cognitive-behavioral psychotherapy: A meta-analysis. *Journal of Consulting and Clinical Psychology* 63:214–220.

Koebnick, C., I. Wagner, P. Leitzmann, U. Stern, and H. J. Zunft. 2003. Probiotic beverage containing *Lactobacillus casei* improves gastrointestinal symptoms in patients with chronic constipation. *Canadian Journal of Gastroenterology.* 17:655–659.

Kohnen, R. and W. D. Oswald. 1988. The effects of valerian, propranolol, and their combination on activation, performance, and mood of healthy volunteers under social stress conditions. *Pharmacopsychiatry* 21:447–4488.

Komatsu, S. 2008. Rice and sushi cravings: A preliminary study of food craving among Japanese females. *Appetite* 50:353–358.

Kris-Etherton, P. M., G. Zhao, A. E. Binkoski, S. M. Coval, and T. D. Etherton. 2001. The effects of nuts on coronary heart disease risk. *Nutrition Reviews* 59(4):103–111.

Kushi, L. H., E. B. Lenart, and W. C. Willett. 1995. Health implications of Mediterranean diets in light of contemporary knowledge, I: Plant foods and dairy products. *American Journal of Clinical Nutrition* 61:1407S–1415S.

Lane, J., J. Seskevich, and C. Pieper. 2007. Brief meditation training can improve perceived stress and negative mood. *Alternative Therapies in Health and Medicine* 13:38–44.

Lappe, J., D. Travers-Gustafson, M. Davies, R. Recker, and R. Heaney. 2007. Vitamin D and calcium supplementation reduces cancer risk: Results of a randomized trial. *American Journal of Clinical Nutrition* 85:1586–1591.

Lawler-Row, K., J. Karremans, C. Scott, M. Edlis-Matityahou, and L. Edwards. 2008. Forgiveness, physiological reactivity, and health: The role of anger. *International Journal of Psychophysiology* 68:51–58.

Lazar, S., G. Bush, R. Gollub, G. Fricchione, G. Khalsa, and H. Benson. 2000. Functional brain mapping of the relaxation response and meditation. *Neuroreport* 11:1581–1585.

Lee, J. K., B. Park, K. Yoo, and Y. Ahn. 1995. Dietary factors and stomach cancer: A case study in Korea. *International Journal of Epidemiology.* 24:33–41

Lemieux, S., D. Prud'homme, C. Bouchard, A. Tremblay, and J. Despres. 1996. A single threshold value of waist girth identifies normal-weight and overweight subjects with excess visceral adipose tissue. *American Journal of Clinical Nutrition* 64:685–693.

Leombruni, P., A. Piero, L. Lavagnino, A. Brustolin, S. Campisi, and S. Fassino. 2008. A randomized, double-blind trial comparing sertraline and fluoxetine 6-month treatment in obese patients with binge eating disorder. *Progress in Neuro-psychopharmacology and Biological Psychiatry* 32(6):1599–1605.

Lilenfeld, L. R., R. Ringham, M. A. Kalarchian, and M. D. Marcus. 2008. A family history study of binge eating disorder. *Comprehensive Psychiatry.* 49(3):247–254.

Linde, K., M. M. Berner, and L. Kriston. 2008. St John's Wort for depression. *Cochrane Database of Systems Reviews* (4):CD00048.

Linehan, M. 1993. *Skills Training Manual for Treating Borderline Personality Disorder.* New York: Guilford Press.

Liu, S., J. Manson, I. Lee, S. Cole, C. Hennekens, W. Willett, and J. Buring. 2000. Fruit and vegetable intake and risk of cardiovascular disease: The Women's Health Study. *American Journal of Clinical Nutrition* 72:922–928.

Lockwood, K., S. Moesgaard, T. Hanioka, and K. Folkers. 1994. Apparent partial remission of breast cancer in "high risk" patients supplemented with nutritional antioxidants, essential fatty acids, and coenzyme Q10. *Molecular Aspects of Medicine* 15:S231–S240.

Logan, A. C. 2004. Omega-3 fatty acids and major depression: A primer for the mental health professional. *Lipids in Health and Disease* 3:25, doi:10.1186/1476-511X-3-25. www.lipidworld.com/content/3/1/25. Accessed January 19, 2009.

Lu, S., H. Lin, K. Lin, and H. Lin. 2008. Quality of life in middle-aged and older Taiwanese patients with rheumatoid arthritis. *Journal of Nursing Research* 16:121–130.

Mackay, N., S. Hansen, and O. McFarlane. 2004. Autonomic nervous system changes during Reiki treatment: A preliminary study. *Journal of Alternative Complementary Medicine* 10:1077–1081.

Maratos, A. S., C. Gold, X. Wang, and M. J. Crawford. 2008. Music therapy for depression. *Cochrane Database Systematic Reviews* 23(1):CD004517, doi: 10.1002/14651858.CD004517.pub2. www.cochrane.org/reviews/en/ab004517.html. Accessed January 19, 2009.

Marcus, M. D. 1997. Adapting treatment for patients with binge eating disorder. In *Handbook of Treatment for Eating Disorders,* second edition, edited by David M. Garner and Paul E. Garfinkel. New York: Guilford Press.

Marcus, M. D., D. Smith, R. Santelli, and W. Kaye. 1992. Characterization of eating disordered behavior in obese binge eaters. *International Journal of Eating Disorders* 12:249–255.

Marcus, M., R. Wing, L. Ewing, E. Kern, W. Gooding, and M. McDermott. 1990. Psychiatric disorders among obese binge eaters. *International Journal of Eating Disorders* 9:69–7.

Masheb, R. M., and C. M. Grilo. 2006. Emotional overeating and its associations with eating disorder psychopathology among overweight patients with binge eating disorder. *International Journal of Eating Disorders* 39(2):141–146.

Matsunaga, M., T. Isowa, K. Kimura, M. Miyakoshi, N. Kanayama, H. Murakami, S. Sato, T. Konagaya, T. Nogimori, S. Fukuyama, J. Shinoda, J. Yamada, and H. Ohira. 2008. Associations among central nervous, endocrine, and immune activities when positive emotions are elicited by looking at a favorite person. *Brain, Behavior, and Immunity* 22(3):408–417.

Mauri, M., P. Rucci, A. Calderone, F. Santini, A. Oppo, A. Romano, S. Rinaldi, A. Armani, M. Polini, A. Pinchera, and G. Cassano. 2008. Axis I and II disorders and quality of life in bariatric surgery candidates. *Journal of Clinical Psychiatry* 69:295–301.

McCullough, M., R. Emmons, and J. Tsang. 2002. The grateful disposition: A conceptual and empirical topography. *Journal of Personality and Social Psychology* 82:112–127.

McElroy, S., J. Hudson, J. Capece, K. Beyers, A. Fisher, and N. Rosenthal. 2007. Topiramate for the treatment of binge eating disorder associated with obesity: A placebo-controlled study. *Biological Psychiatry* 61:1039–1048.

Middlekauff, H., J. L. Yu, and K. Hui. 2001. Acupuncture effects on reflex responses to mental stress in humans. *American Journal Physiology Regulatory Integrative Comparative Physiology* 280:R1462–R1468

Milano, W., C. Petrella, A. Casella, A. Capasso, S. Carrino, and L. Milano. 2005. Use of sibutramine, an inhibitor of the reuptake of serotonin and noradrenaline, in the treatment of binge eating disorder: A placebo-controlled study. *Advances in Therapy* 22(1):25–31.

Mills, D. E., K. M. Prkachin, K. A. Harvey, and R. P. Ward. 1989. Dietary fatty acid supplementation alters stress reactivity and performance in man. *Journal of Human Hypertension* 3:111–116.

Mills, S. and K. Bone. 2000. Ginseng. In *Principles and Practice of Phytotherapy: Modern Herbal Medicine.* New York: Churchill Livingstone.

Mitchell, K. S., and S. E. Mazzeo. 2004. Binge eating and psychological distress in ethnically diverse undergraduate men and women. *Eating Behaviors* 5(2):157–169.

Murphy, G. E., R. M. Carney, M. A. Knesevich, R. D. Wetzel, and P. Whitworth. 1995. Cognitive behavior therapy, relaxation training, and tricyclic antidepressant medication in the treatment of depression. *Psychology Reports* 77(2):403–420.

National Center for Complementary and Alternative Medicine. 2004. *Manipulative and Body-Based Practices: An Overview.* Bethesda, MD: National Center for Complementary and Alternative Medicine.

National Institutes of Health. 1998. *The Clinical Guidelines on the Identification, Evaluation, and Treatment of Overweight and Obesity in Adults: The Evidence Report.* NIH Publications. www.nhlbi.nih.gov /guidelines/obesity/e_txtbk/index.htm. Accessed January 19, 2009.

NIH Backgrounder. 2002. Stress system malfunction could lead to serious, life threatening disease. www .nih.gov/news/pr/sep2002/nichd-09.htm. Accessed January 16, 2009.

O'Brien, C., A. Childress, R. Ehrman, and S. Robbins. 1998. Conditioning factors in drug abuse: Can they explain compulsion? *Journal of Psychopharmacology* 12:15–22.

Office of Dietary Supplements. Dietary supplement fact sheets. ods.od.nih.gov/factsheets. Accessed November 14, 2008.

Office of the Surgeon General. 1996. Physical activity and health. Retrieved www.surgeongeneral.gov /library/reports/index.html. Accessed October 29, 2008.

Paluska, S. A., and T. L. Schwenk. 2000. Physical activity and mental health: Current concepts. *Sports Medicine* 29(3):167–180.

Petry, N. M., D. Barry, R. H. Pietrzak, and J. A. Wagner. 2007. Overweight and obesity are associated with psychiatric disorders: Results from the national epidemiologic survey on alcohol and related conditions. *Psychosomatic Medicine* 70(3):288–297.

Picot, A., and L. Lilenfeld. 2003. The relationship among binge severity, personality psychopathology, and body mass index. *International Journal of Eating Disorders* 34:98–107.

Pittas, A., P. Lau, F. Hu, and B. Dawson. 2007. The role of vitamin D and calcium in type 2 diabetes: A systematic review and meta-analysis. *Journal of Clinical Endocrinology and Metabolism* 92(6):2017-2029.

Poldinger, W., B. Calanchini, and W. Schwarz. 1991. A functional-dimensional approach to depression: Serotonin deficiency as a target syndrome in a comparison of 5- hydroxytryptophan and fluvoxamine. *Psychopathology* 24:53–81.

Pop-Jordanova, N. 2000. Psychological characteristics and biofeedback mitigation in preadolescents with eating disorders. *Pediatrics International* 42:76–81.

Popkess-Vawter, S., E. Yoder, and B. Gajewski. 2005. The role of spirituality in holistic weight management. *Clinical Nursing Research* 14:158–174.

Pull, C. P. 2004. Binge eating disorder. *Current Opinion Psychiatry* 17:43–48.

Rayworth, B. B., L. A. Wise, and B. L. Harlow. 2004. Childhood abuse and risk of eating disorders in women. *Epidemiology* 15(3):271–278.

Reas, D., and C. Grilo. 2008. Review and meta-analysis of pharmacotherapy for binge eating disorder. *Obesity* 16(9):2024–2038.

Reicks, M., J. Mills, and H. Henry. 2004. Qualitative study of spirituality in a weight loss program: Contribution to self-efficacy and locus of control. *Journal of Nutrition Education Behavior* 36:13–15.

Reynolds, W., and K. Coats. 1986. A comparison of cognitive-behavioral therapy and relaxation training for the treatment of depression in adolescents. *Journal of Consulting Clinical Psychology* 54:653–660.

Richards, S., M. Berrett, R. Hardman, and D. Eggett. 2006. Comparative efficacy of spirituality, cognitive, and emotional support groups for treating eating disorder inpatients. *Eating Disorders* 14:401–415.

Rosenbaum, J. F., M. Fava, W. E. Falk, M. H. Pollack, L. S. Cohen, B. M. Cohen, and G. S. Zubenko. 2007. The antidepressant potential of oral S-adenosyl-l-methionine. *Acta Psychiatrica Scandinavica* 81(5):432–436.

Rosenkranz, M., D. Jackson, K. Dalton, I. Dolski, C. Ryff, B. Singer, D. Muller, N. Kalin, and R. Davidson. 2003. Affective style and in vivo immune response: Neurobehavioral mechanisms. *Proceedings of the National Academy of Sciences* 100:11148–11152

Ross, C. 2007. *Healing Body, Mind and Spirit: An Integrative Medicine Approach to the Treatment of Eating Disorders.* Denver, CO: Outskirts Press.

Ross, C., P. M. Herman, O. Rocklin, and J. Rojas. 2008. Evaluation of integrative medicine for eating disorders. *Explore: The Journal of Science and Healing* 4(5):315–320.

Ross, C., R. D. Langer, and E. Barrett-Conner. 1997. Given diabetes: Is fat better than thin? *Diabetes Care* 20:650–652.

Ross, C. C. 2007. Qigong. In *Complementary and Alternative Treatments in Mental Health Care*, edited by J. Lake and D. Spiegel. Washington, D.C.: American Psychiatric Publishing, Inc.

Sanchez-Castillo, C., O. Velazquez-Monroy, A. Berber, A. Lara-Esqueda, R. Tapia-Conyer, and P. James. 2003. Anthropometric cutoff points for predicting chronic diseases in the Mexican National Health Survey 2000. *Obesity Research* 11:442–451.

Sanders, M. 2000. Considerations for use of probiotic bacteria to modulate human health. *Journal of Nutrition* 130:384S–390S

Schruers, K., H. Pols, and T. Overbeek. 2002. Acute L-5-hydroxytryptophan administration inhibits carbon dioxide–induced panic in panic disorder patients. *Psychiatry Research* 113(3):237–243.

Scragg, R., M. Sowers, and C. Bell. 2007. Serum 25-hydroxyvitamin D, ethnicity, and blood pressure in the Third National Health and Nutrition Examination Survey. *American Journal of Hypertension* 20:713–719.

Selye, H. 1976. Forty years of stress research: Principal remaining problems and misconceptions. *Canadian Medical Association Journal* 115(1):53–56.

Shade, E., C. Ulrich, M. Wener, B. Wood, Y. Yasui, K. Lacroix, J. Potter, and A. McTiernan. 2004. Frequent intentional weight loss is associated with lower natural killer cell cytotoxicity in post-menopausal women: Possible long-term immune effects. *Journal of the American Dietetic Association* 104:903–912.

Shaw, K., J. Turner, and C. Del Mar. 2002. Tryptophan and 5-hydroxytryptophan for depression. *Cochrane Database System Reviews* 1:CD003198, doi:10.1002/14651858. CD003198. www.cochrane.org/reviews /en/ab003198.html. Accessed January 19, 2009.

Shore, A. 2004. Long-term effects of energetic healing on symptoms of psychological depression and self-perceived stress. *Alternative Therapy Health Medicine* 10:42–48.

Simpson, D. and M. P. Curran. 2008. Ramelteon: A review of its use in insomnia. *Drugs* 68(13):1901–1919.

Siple, M. 1999. *Healing Food for Dummies*. IDG Books Worldwide, Inc. Foster City, CA.

Smith, C. A. and P. P. Hay. 2005. Acupuncture for depression. *Cochrane Database System Reviews* 18:70–76.

Smyth, J. M., K. E. Heron, S. A. Wonderlich, R. D. Crosby, and K. M. Thompson. 2008. The influence of reported trauma and adverse events on eating disturbance in young adults. *International Journal of Eating Disorders* 41(3):195–202.

Somer, E. 1999. *Food and Mood: The Complete Guide to Eating Well and Feeling Your Best*. New York: Henry Holt and Company.

Sorensen, H., and J. Sonne. 1996. A double-masked study of the effects of ginseng on cognitive functions. *Current Therapy Research* 57:959–968.

Sotaniemi, E. A., E. Haapakoski, and A. Rautio. 1995. Ginseng therapy in non-insulin dependent diabetic patients. *Diabetes Care* 18:1373–1375.

Specker, S., M. de Zwaan, N. Raymond, and J. Mitchell. 1994. Psychopathology in subgroups of obese women with and without binge eating disorder. *Comparative Psychiatry* 35:185–190.

Spitzer, R. L., S. Yanovski, T. Wadden, R. Wing, M. D. Marcus, A. Stunkard, M. Devlin, J. Mitchell, D. Hasin, and R. L. Horne. 1993. Binge eating disorder: Its further validation in a multi-site study. *International Journal of Eating Disorders* 13:137–153.

Stice, E., K. Presnell, and D. Spangler. 2002. Risk factors for binge eating onset in adolescent girls: A two-year prospective investigation. *Health Psychology* 2:131–138.

Striegel-Moore, R., F. A. Dohm, K. Pike, D. Wilfley, and C. Fairburn. 2002. Abuse, bullying, and discrimination as risk factors for binge eating disorder. *American Journal of Psychiatry* 159:1902–1907.

Stunkard, A. 2004. Binge eating disorder and the night-eating syndrome. In *Handbook of Obesity Treatment*. ed. T. Wadden and A. Stunkard. New York: The Guilford Press.

Stunkard, A. J., M. Fernstrom, A. Price, E. Frank, and D. Kupfer. 1990. Direction of weight gain in recurrent depression: Consistency across episodes. *Archives of General Psychiatry* 47:857–860.

Stunkard, A. J., J. R. Harris, N. L. Pedersen, and G. E. McClearn. 1990. The body mass index of twins who have been reared apart. *New England Journal of Medicine* 322:1483–1487.

Sublette, M. E., J. R. Hibbeln, H. Galfalvy, M. Oquendo, and J. J. Mann. 2006. Omega-3 polyunsaturated essential fatty acid status as a predictor of future suicide risk. *American Journal of Psychiatry* 163:1100–1102.

Tang, B., G. Eslick, C. Nowson, C. Smith, and A. Bensoussan. 2007. Use of calcium or calcium in combination with vitamin D supplementation to prevent fractures and bone loss in people aged 50 years and older: A meta-analysis. *Lancet* 370(9588):657–666.

Tang, Y., Y. Ma, J. Wang, Y. Fan, S. Feng, Q. Lu, Q. Yu, D. Sui, M. Rothbart, M. Fan, and M. Posner. 2007. Short-term meditation training improves attention and self-regulation. *Proceedings of the National Academy of Science* 104:17152–17156.

Taylor, M., S. Carney, G. Goodwin, and J. Geddes. 2003. Folate for depressive disorders. *Cochrane Database of Systematic Reviews* 2:CD003390, doi: 10.1002/14651858.CD003390. www.cochrane.org/reviews/en/ab003390.html. Accessed January 19, 2009.

Taylor, L. H., and K. A. Kobak. 2000. An open-label trial of St. John's wort (*Hypericum perforatum*) in obsessive-compulsive disorder. *Journal of Clinical Psychiatry* 61:575–578.

Telch, C. F., W. S. Agras, and M. M. Linehan. 2001. Dialectical behavior therapy for binge eating disorder. *Journal of Consulting and Clinical Psychology* 69:1061–1065.

Tobin, D. L., A. L. Molteni, and M. R. Elin. 1995. Early trauma, dissociation, and late onset in eating disorders. *International Journal of Eating Disorders* 17(3):305–308.

Tuck, I., R. Alleyne, and W. Thinganjana. 2006. Spirituality and stress management in healthy adults. *Journal of Holistic Nursing* 24:245–253.

Tucker, K. L., S. Rich, I. Rosenberg, P. Jacques, G. Dallal, W. F. Wilson, and J. Selhub. 2000. Plasma vitamin B12 concentrations relate to intake source in the Framingham Offspring Study. *American Journal of Clinical Nutrition* 71:514–522.

Turk, D., K. Swanson, and E. Tunks. 2008. Psychological approaches in the treatment of chronic pain patients: When pills, scalpels and needles are not enough. *Canadian Journal of Psychiatry* 53:212–223.

Turnbaugh, P., R. Ley, M. Mahowald, V. Magrini, E. Mardis, and J. Gordon. 2006. An obesity-associated gut microbiome with increased capacity for energy harvest. *Nature* 444:1027–1031.

Tuthill, A, H. Slawik, S. O'Rahilly, and N. Finer. 2006. Psychiatric co-morbidities in patients attending specialist obesity services in the UK. *Quarterly Journal of Medicine* 99:317–325.

Uher, R., T. Murphy, M. Brammer, T. Dalgleish, M. Phillips, W. Ng, A. C. Virginia, S. Williams, I. Campbell, and J. Treasure. 2004. Medial prefrontal cortex activity associated with symptom provocation in eating disorders. *American Journal of Psychiatry* 161:1238–1246.

Van Dongen, H. P. A., G. Maislin, J. M. Mullington, and D. F. Dinges. 2003. The cumulative cost of additional wakefulness: Dose-response effects on neurobehavioral functions and sleep physiology from chronic sleep restriction and total sleep deprivation. *Sleep* 26(2):117–126.

Van Praag, H. M. 1996. Faulty cortisol/serotonin interplay. Psychopathological and biological characterisation of a new, hypothetical depression subtype (SeCA depression). *Psychiatry Research* 65(3):143–157.

———. 2002. Crossroads of corticotropin releasing hormone, corticosteroids and monoamines. About a biological interface between stress and depression. *Neurotoxicity Research* 4(5–6):531–555.

———. 2005. Can stress cause depression? *The World Journal of Biological Psychiatry* 6(2):5–22.

Vanitallie, T. B. 2002. Stress: A risk factor for serious illness. *Metabolism* 51(6, 1):40–45.

Vieweg, W. V., D. A. Julius, J. Bates, J. F. Quinn 3rd, A. Fernandez, M. Hasnain, and A. K. Pandurangi. 2007. Posttraumatic stress disorder as a risk factor for obesity among male military veterans. *Acta Psychiatrica Scandinavica* 116(6):483–487.

Visscher, T. L. S., J. C. Seidell, A. Molarius, D. van der Kuip, A. Hofman, and J. C. M. Witteman. 2001. A comparison of body mass index, waist-hip ratio, and waist circumference as predictors of all-cause mortality among the elderly: The Rotterdam study. *International Journal of Obesity.* 25:1730–1735.

Vgontzas, A. N., E. O. Bixler, G. P. Chrousos, and S. Pejovic. 2008. Obesity and sleep disturbances: Meaningful sub-typing of obesity. *Archives of Physiology and Biochemistry* 114(4):224–236.

Walsh, B. 2008. Hypnotic alteration of body image in the eating disordered. *American Journal of Clinical Hypnosis* 50:301–310.

Walsh, T., and G. Boudreau. 2003. Laboratory studies of binge eating disorder. *International Journal of Eating Disorders* 34(Suppl):30–38.

WebMD. 2008. Sleep 101. *Medscape Neurology & Neurosurgery.* www.medscape.com/viewarticle/578698. Accessed September 22, 2008.

Webster, M. J. 1998. Physiological and performance responses to supplementation with thiamin and pantothenic acid derivatives. *European Journal of Applied Physiology and Occupational Physiology* 77:486–491.

Weissenburger, J., J. Rush, D. Gilles, and A. Stunkard. 1986. Weight change in depression. *Psychiatry Research* 17:275–283.

Wheatley, D. 2001. Kava and valerian in the treatment of stress-induced insomnia. *Phytotherapy Research.* 15(6):549–551.

Wildman, R. P., D. Gu, K. Reynolds, X. Duan, and J. He. 2004. Appropriate body mass index and waist circumference cutoffs for categorization of overweight and central adiposity among Chinese adults. *American Journal of Clinical Nutrition.* 80:1129–1136.

Wilfley, D. E., J. C. Scott, J. I. Hudson, J. E. Mitchell, R. I. Berkowitz, V. Blakesley, and B. T. Walsh. 2008. Efficacy of sibutramine for the treatment of binge eating disorder: A randomized multicenter placebo-controlled double-blind study. *American Journal of Psychiatry* 165:51–58.

Wilfley, D. E., S. Agras, C. Telch, E. Rossiter, J. Schneider, A. G. Cole, L. Sifford, and S. Raeburn. 1993. Group cognitive-behavioural therapy and group interpersonal psychotherapy for the non-purging bulimic individual: A controlled comparison. *Journal of Consulting and Clinical Psychology* 61:296–305

Wilson, T., A. Milosevic, M. Carroll, K. Hart, and S. Hibbard. 2008. Physical health status in relation to self-forgiveness and other-forgiveness in healthy college students. *Journal of Health Psychology* 13:798–803.

Winstead-Fry, P., and J. Kijek. An integrative review and meta-analysis of therapeutic touch research. *Alternative Therapies in Health and Medicine* 5:58–67.

Wollowski, I., G. Rechkemmer, and B. Pool-Zobel. 2001. Protective role of probiotics and prebiotics in colon cancer. *American Journal of Clinical Nutrition* 73:451S–455S.

Wortsman, J., L. Matsuoka, T. Chen, Z. Lu, and M. Holick. 2000. Decreased bioavailability of vitamin D in obesity. *American Journal of Clinical Nutrition* 72:690–693.

Yanovski, S. Z. 1993. Binge eating disorder: Current knowledge and future directions. *Obesity Research* 1(4):306–324.

Zakarian, J., M. Hovellm, T. Conway, R. Hofstetter, and D. Slymen. 2000. Tobacco use and other risk behaviors: Cross-sectional and predictive relationships for adolescent orthodontic patients. *Nicotine and Tobacco Research* 2:179–186.

Zanarini, M., and F. Frankenburt. 2003. Omega-3 fatty acid treatment of women with borderline personality disorder: A double-blind, placebo-controlled pilot study. *American Journal of Psychiatry* 160:167–169.

Zand, J. 1999. The natural pharmacy: Herbal medicine for depression. In *Natural Healing for Depression: Solutions from the World's Great Health Traditions and Practitioners*, ed. J. Strohecker and N. S. Strohecker. New York:Penguin-Putnam.

Zellner, D. A., S. Loaiza, Z. Gonzalez, J. Pita, J. Morales, D. Pecora, and A. Wolf. 2006. Food selection changes under stress. *Physiology and Behavior* 87(4):789–793.

Zung, W. 1965. A self-rating depression scale. *Archives of General Psychiatry* vol. 63–70.

———. 1971. A rating instrument for anxiety. *Psychosomatics* 12:371–379.

Carolyn Coker Ross, MD, MPH, is a physician, author, and nationally recognized speaker. Ross is a graduate of the University of Michigan Medical School and an alumna of Andrew Weil's integrative medicine program at the University of Arizona. She is board-certified in addiction medicine. She is former chief of the eating disorders program at Sierra Tucson, an addiction treatment center in Tucson, AZ. She is currently in private practice in Denver, CO, and is a consultant for eating disorder and chemical dependency treatment centers nationally.

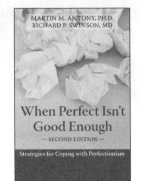
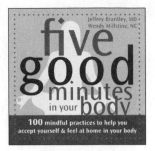
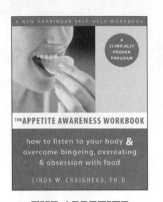
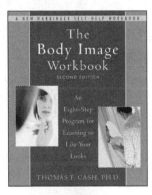
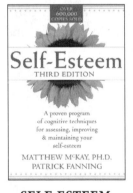
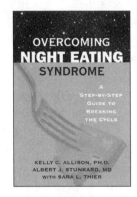
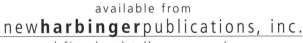